The Relativity Diet

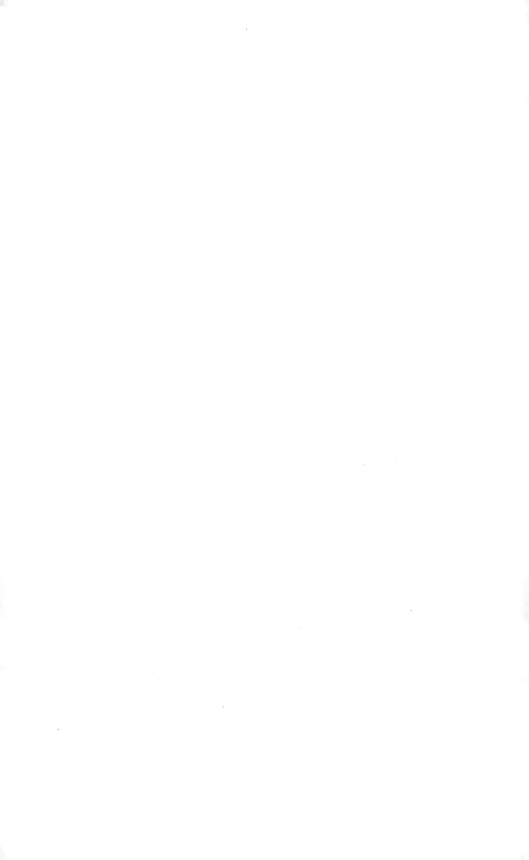

The Relativity Diet

A DIET THEORY OF EVERYTHING

SHAUN J. MELARVIE, M.D.

EVENT HORIZON PUBLISHING

The Relativity Diet:
A Diet Theory of Everything
by Shaun J. Melarvie, M.D.
author@relativitydiet.com

Published by:
Event Horizon Publishing
PO Box 609
Sturgeon Bay, Wisconsin 54235-0609
(920) 559-0269
info@eventhorizonpublishing.com
www.eventhorizonpublishing.com

The photograph on page 45 is © Geronimo / Fotolia. The photograph on page 47 is © Petro Feketa / Fotolia. The cartoons on pages 201, 202, 204, and 264 are © Ruth Brendemuehl. The photograph on page 336 is © Julie Wohlberg / Fotolia.

Nothing in *The Relativity Diet: A Diet Theory of Everything* should be construed as an attempt to offer or render a medical opinion or otherwise engage in the practice of medicine. The medical information provided herein is of a general nature and cannot substitute for the patient-specific advice of a medical professional. Please seek the advice of a qualified medical professional before following any practice, diet, or program discussed in this book.

ISBN: 978-0-9841872-4-9
LCCN: 2009934624

Design and composition: www.dmargulis.com

Manufactured in the United States of America

Whatever you can do or dream you can, begin it.
Boldness has genius, power, and magic in it.

Goethe

for Susan, *always*

Contents

Dear Reader,

I am inviting you on a personal journey of discovery in the pages that follow. You will learn much, you will laugh often, and you will feel sadness only rarely. It is my belief that along the way you will undergo a process of self-actualization that will culminate in a changed perspective of your true place in the universe—a happier and healthier place.

There are two primary reasons to read this book: if you are unhappy, or if you are overweight or obese. And if you are both, you'd better have a glass of water, find a quiet place, and start reading right now. As you are probably aware, we are in the midst of a worldwide epidemic of obesity. Overweight and obesity have become so common that to be so is almost considered normal. With such a focus on the collective problem of obesity, it is easy to lose sight of the fact that it is not so much a collective problem as it is a deeply personal one.

I have approached obesity as the personal war that it is. I have pulled back the curtain to expose the misperceptions, half-truths, and outright lies that feed this monster we call obesity. I will reveal all that is pertinent to weight loss, all that matters, and that which does not. You will find that I often speak in absolutes in my efforts to impress upon you the significance of what I am relating. I realize there is more nuance, but nuance can be confusing, and I want no confusion.

The problem with most weight loss approaches is that they are focused solely on how to change how you eat. I am focused on how to change how you think, and if we can accomplish that, everything else will follow. All that you will read in these pages is evidence-based and true to the natural laws of our universe: this is my solemn promise to you.

The Relativity Diet is a story of truth and science that will be as a stone of empowerment with which you will slay the Goliath of obesity. It is meant to be read as you would a story, in a leisurely fashion, with no effort to remember *this* or write down *that*, because it is all summarized for you at the end. *The Relativity Diet* is a hybrid of science and narrative that is best experienced in continuity the first time. So sit back, relax, and enjoy—just start at the beginning; read through the middle; and when you get to the end, don't stop—for you are just beginning.

It is time.

Shaun

Shaun Melarvie

Sturgeon Bay, Wisconsin
January 2010

Acknowledgments

LTHOUGH WRITING IS LARGELY a solitary effort, with much time spent alone pondering the use of a compound sentence or the dissonance of *subliminally* in a prepositional phrase, there is an unseen infrastructure that makes everything possible. It is this infrastructure that is the content of acknowledgment sections found in most books, and *The Relativity Diet* is no exception.

I would like to start with both an apology and an appreciation to my very first readers, Kathy Rowe, Vivian Fink, and Mike Bruno: an appreciation for suffering through my first effort of sixty thousand words; and an apology for the fact that few of those words survived the final effort of ninety thousand. However, it was because of their input that I was able to better focus my message in a more meaningful way. I am grateful for the tolerance my co-workers at Door County Memorial Hospital demonstrated over the course of hundreds of colonoscopies during which I experimented with my prose; and an extra thanks for a few who managed to make appearances in the aforementioned prose. There is a surgical technician who I work with most days of the week. Lucky for me, she also happens to be an artist and managed to turn my stick drawings into usable illustrations, which she signs as Ruth Brendemuehl. I must thank Deb Knippel of Ministry Healthcare for her kind and efficient assistance with my review of numerous journal articles.

There is a man of science, a physicist, who took the time to guide me through the absurdity of quantum theory, while at the same time gently illuminating my ignorance. Thank you. I am indebted to Carmen Schroeder, R.D., C.D., C.D.E., for her professional assistance with the nutritional aspects of my book and her kind tolerance of my repeated phone calls. Linda Ferrari endured my longest effort and was responsible for a two-thousand-word haircut of the section, during which she had the audacity to nod off, no matter how many times she read it.

Norbert Blei, author, poet, publisher, friend: thank you, Norb, for that winter morn, after the storm, at DC Coffee. It was your kind critique that lent the encouragement to bring my work down the homestretch. I remembered when I called you three years earlier, and I am glad that you did not read what I had written then. Dick Margulis designed and produced the book as well as educating me about the mechanics of publishing. Katharine Wiencke proofread the pages, contributing many valuable suggestions. The book is much improved for their help. Any remaining errors in the book are, of course, entirely my responsibility.

Lastly, as you will come to discover, none of this would have been possible without the love, support, and inspiration of my beautiful and talented wife of twenty-five years. She has been a reader, but more importantly, a listener: many a night I would print a passage that I had been working on so I could read it to her. Thank you, dear, for posting the note on my monitor that got me started. I have also enjoyed the counsel and support of my children: Jason, Eric, Jessica, and Shaun.

The problem with an acknowledgments section is that once you start, it is difficult to stop, because a series of actions that culminates in a finished work is only the cumulative product of life experiences. There are many friends, acquaintances, teachers, and relatives who have significantly affected my life-product; therefore, to all I know, thank you.

The Relativity Diet

PRE-ENLIGHTENMENT

What a piece of work is a man
how infinite in faculties,
in form and moving how express and admirable,
in action how like an angel,
in apprehension how like a god!
the beauty of the world,
the paragon of animals—and yet,
to me, what is this quintessence of dust?

W. Shakespeare

chapter one

A brief history of my obesity

1961–2004

NEVER WAS LITTLE. I never had a growth spurt, shooting up over the course of the summer—I always was about as big at the end of the school term as I was at the start of the next one, relative to my peers. From the day I was born at twelve pounds to the peak of my obesity some forty years later at over three hundred, my body mass remained on a steady upwards trajectory but for one brief interruption brought on by the happy coincidence of adolescence and testosterone. As of September twenty-first, 1961, I was the largest baby ever born in the Prairie du Chien Memorial Hospital. A long labor, before the era of epidurals and high C-section rates, left me with a misshapen head from the forceps that pulled me headfirst from my mother's birth canal. I was nearly twice as large as any other baby in the viewing window and as I banged away on the sides of an ill-fitting bassinet people pointed at me and exclaimed something to the effect of *ooh, what a huge baby… what's wrong with the poor thing… look at his head, it's shaped like a heart.* My father told me years later that when asked if I was his baby he replied that no, *it was not*—he denied me if not three times, at least once.

Other than my size, my years in elementary school were only remarkable for my shyness due to some initial difficulty in first grade with the proper use of articles in sentence structure. I often circled an *a* when I should have circled an *an*, which caused Mrs. Gussman much consternation. She'd circle my incorrect selections with a heavy red marker that everybody else could see when she passed back the papers. I'm not sure what happened to me that summer between first and second grade; all I know is that my new teacher, Mrs. Morris, wasn't nearly so consternated, I didn't see so much red and I began to do better.

My steadily increasing height and weight spared me from the taunts and abuses of bullies from within my peer group and those early years were largely stress free and I was quite happy to be bigger than everyone else. Then one day I graduated from recess to physical education. For the first time in my life, I found my size to be a detriment. I couldn't run as fast or jump as high as most others, and for some inexplicable reason, I could not hit a ball with a bat. I avoided all physical activity I could that involved group competition where other children might have to count on my performance. After school and on the weekends, my preference was not playing softball or any other team sport outside. My preference was taking refuge in the overstuffed La-Z-Boy recliner in our living room and reading something along the lines of *The Hardy Boys and the Secret of Wildcat Swamp*, or *Tarzan and the Jewels of Opar* or, better yet, *Slave Girl of Gor*, because of the picture of an almost naked slave girl on the cover.

Late in the summer, my mother would take me to Sears Roebuck to get clothes for school. This was in the seventies, long before PlayStation and the iPod, when most kids spent their time outside rather than in front of an LCD screen. The store would be filled with mothers with children in tow, and I remember feeling nervous, shy, and embarrassed, all at the same time.

The summer we moved to Bismarck, North Dakota I was entering fifth grade at a new public school, Walker Junior High. My mother, a product of parochial schools, who never missed a day of church in her life, called it "The Jungle." She imagined drug dealers on the corner and sex acts performed under desks while the teacher, most likely a devil worshiper, took unauthorized breaks in a smoke-filled back room.

As usual, my straight-line growth from the previous year necessitated a trip to Sears with my mother to properly outfit me for the pending toils of fifth grade in the jungle. It was important for her to have me well clothed, including a fresh supply of whitey-tighties. She selected my various vestments with as much care as if they were a suit of armor that would protect me from the arrows of immorality that were sure to be launched from the dark satanic recesses of Walker Junior High—that towering brick edifice that clutched at her heart with icy fingers of foreboding every time she passed it by.

Back then I don't remember there being much variety in jeans, like "relaxed-fit," "loose-fit," "standard," "easy-fit," or "slim-cut." I think that all they had were "slim," "regular," and "husky," which I never took notice of before. I knew that I was *thicker* than most of my friends, but I never really thought of myself as being *husky,* at least not until my fifth grade year.

It always took Mom a few minutes to find the husky sizes. They were invariably to the right on the rack and on the bottom of the piles. "Sizes for a boy who needs a fuller fit" the sign said, not as discreetly as I would have hoped.

"Here, Shaun, try these on," she said, handing me a pair of Wranglers pulled from the bottom of a pile.

"Okay." In the dressing room I slipped out of the soft denim, with the knee patches my grandmother had sewn on, and into the stiff, new jeans. They felt like cardboard; I couldn't imagine them ever being comfortable.

"Well? Shaun?"

"Coming, Mom." I stepped out of the changing room and stood at attention for her inspection.

"Not bad," she said, assessing the length. She rolled up the cuffs that would allow an additional two-inch increase in height.

"How do they feel?" she asked.

"Okay." I didn't tell her the part about them feeling like cardboard. I knew what was coming next. I looked around to see if anyone was watching.

"Now turn around." As I turned around she stuck her fingers inside the waist above my butt and gave a good tug, making sure she had about four finger breadths of space. She did, because, in order for the jeans to accommodate my buttocks, the waist needed to be much bigger than was necessary.

"They look really nice, Shaun." She smiled and asked, "Do you like them?"

"Sure, Mom," I said. "Thanks."

Shirts, socks, and underwear were relatively pain-less since there wasn't the need for so much hands-on evaluating; regrettably, shoes were a different story. Shoes during this period of my life didn't hold much variety. The common denominators were the three *B's*: *big, brown,* and *boxy*—oh, and *suede*. I suppose that would be the "*s*" after the apostrophe.

"These look nice." Mom held out a pair of brown suede shoes that looked strangely like newer versions of what I was wearing, only bigger.

A shoe salesman materialized out of thin air. Before I could say *what about those dingo boots,* he had me laced up and standing in front of my mother, who dropped to her knees rather naturally, given her regular church attendance. She buried her right thumb into the empty suede pocket immediately in front of my big toe.

"These seem to fit." She breathed a small sigh of satisfaction, noticing the potential for further growth. "How do they feel, Shaun?"

"Fine, Mom." As she stood up I wiggled my big toe to pop out the dent that her thumb had made.

This maneuver was repeated in the routine fashion a second time for a pair of canvas tennis shoes with crescent moon, rubberized tips. Each time my mother genuflected, I self-consciously scanned my immediate surroundings. As in most cases, my emotional distress was largely self-inflicted—all of my peers, scattered around the store, were too wrapped up in their own worlds to be interested in mine.

I love my mother tremendously, and she sized me up for jeans and footwear through the first year of high school. Although I was embarrassed to have her so involved in my clothing process, I didn't want to hurt her feelings; after all, she *was* paying for them. I felt that I owed it to her—the *satisfaction of a good fit for her not-so-little boy.* By the time I was sixteen, I had a job and was buying my clothes for myself. Thank God.

Somewhere between ninth and tenth grade my huskiness left me, momentarily, quite by accident. This happy occurrence was related more to the metabolism of an adolescent and an increase in energy expenditure, rather than any attention, whatsoever, paid to my diet. Like most adolescent males, I wanted to be a chick magnet. The general idea was that this involved a nice car, the ability to kick some ass, and lots of muscles. Intelligence and sensitivity were assigned a much lower value on the male adolescent scale of desirability.

I acquired a cobalt blue, 1970 Dodge Challenger with bucket seats and white racing stripes down the sides—check. My best friend and I joined a Tae Kwon Do class, watched every Bruce Lee and Chuck Norris movie ever made, and practiced intricately lethal kung fu moves on each other in slow motion—check. I joined track; since I could only run eight-minute miles, I threw the shot put, discus, and javelin instead—check. By the time of my senior year in high school I was fairly close to the Greek ideal of the male physical form, and if not an athletic star, at least I found myself in the near vicinity of athletic stars.

But the one thing I couldn't participate in was football, because of a head injury I sustained as a child, and all my life long I had the impression of a missed opportunity. I remember one afternoon at Dan's Supervalu, where I worked as a carryout, an older gentleman who must have been a St. Mary's High School Booster asked me if I played football. I was wearing a pair of slinky black disco slacks that hugged my hips and a baby-blue tee-shirt with "Supervalu Days" emblazoned on the front. I told the gentleman that I couldn't play contact sports because of a head injury.

He shook his head back and forth. "Tsk, tsk, tsk, what a waste of a body," he said, which pretty much summed up my feelings as well. I asked my dad after supper that night if I could join the football team. I got the same answer as the last time I asked.

Although I was in possession of the aforementioned qualities, I never did become a chick magnet because, as it turned out, I was afraid of girls. I couldn't talk to them and was convinced that they found me unsightly. I didn't realize at the time that I vaguely resembled the young Lord Greystoke of Edgar Rice Burroughs fame whom I had spent so many hours with in the La-Z-Boy. It was only years later as a hopelessly obese and dysfunctional adult that I realized this while flipping through faded photographs. *If only I could have played football.*

The absolute nadir of my adult weight occurred during my summer of Army advanced individual training for the North Dakota Army National Guard in 1984. I was twenty-two years old, six feet, three inches tall, and weighed one hundred and eighty-six pounds, which is a body mass index (BMI) of 23 (healthy weight). Twenty years later I was six feet, three inches tall and weighed three hundred pounds, which is a BMI approaching forty, which meant that I was morbidly obese. This is when my life changed. I think of it as my awakening and it started in the New Year.

considering that I exercised somewhat regularly during this period of time, I would have to admit that this may not have been out of line with my refined sugar intake.

Was I just hungry? You bet I was. I was hungry for something, and I interpreted the emptiness that needed filling as hunger, and I ate. I ate big meals of two to three servings, sometimes more, and I ate big snacks between my big meals. Much of the time I wasn't looking for it, but if it presented itself to me, such as a tray of cookies in a staff lounge or at a noon meeting, I ate it, or, more correctly, I ate them, because one or two were never enough.

In the middle of the second week of December my wife hosted a mitten-making party. She had six friends over to show them how to make woolen mittens from old sweaters that she had picked up at Goodwill. Ironically, only two weeks before she had acquired this skill we had taken three plastic garbage bags stuffed with woolen sweaters to the very same Goodwill store. It is almost certain that Sue bought back at least one of those sweaters—I mean, if she was drawn to a certain color or pattern the first time, why not a second time as well.

The ladies walked through our front door that chilly December evening one at a time, and with them came a total of six multiple servings of fudge, cookies, brownies, and other things sweet. Sue had her own contributions settled about the house. One of her contributions was what I assumed were foil-wrapped hard candies. I was happy that I found these in the center of the bar table in my office—happy because I didn't care for hard candies and it would be easy for me to resist eating them as opposed to a plate of fudge, for instance.

I occupied myself in the office with our annual Christmas letter while in the background female voices drifted into my consciousness, "Oh, my God. That is just darling!"

"This is so easy. I'm going to make tiny pairs for all my nieces."

"What wonderful eggnog, Sue."

I nod in silent agreement, licking a creamy mustache from my upper lip. The sewing room is at the end of the bonus room that branches perpendicularly from the back of my office, so the women are just around the corner—unseen but not unheard; out of sight but not out of mind. It is of no matter; I have other fish to fry tonight.

I find myself sitting at the bar table, twirling a red-foiled candy between my fingers, trapped in a transient writer's block, wondering if the words *morning heat bolus* and *septic tank* would be appropriate for my Christmas letter. For some reason, I peel off the red foil. I am pleasantly surprised to discover a milk chocolate truffle rather than the red-and-white-striped hard candy I had been expecting and couldn't stand. I never liked mint. The only mints I would ever eat were the chocolate-covered ones that I'd suffer through in a box of candies, in the hopes of finding the kind that I really liked—soft, chocolate, chewy, caramel fudge, with the only crunch being that from nuts.

Hmmm? I bite the truffle in half. I am gratified to find a rich, creamy, softer chocolate center, with a hint of... amaretto or cherry? It's hard to say. The thick creamy texture coats the mucosal membranes of my mouth. I mash the soft chocolate between my tongue and hard palate. Chocolate stimulates my taste buds, telling the pleasure center of my cerebral cortex that it is a good thing. I slide my tongue back and forth and from side to side, sucking the adherent layer of melted chocolate from the inside of my mouth, and swallow. It is this finishing act of muscular contraction in the back of my throat that completes the pleasure cycle. It is as a sexual emission; all before it is mere foreplay.

I must swallow. I cannot fathom tasting and spitting, like wine, but, then, I don't spit wine either. How nice it would be if I could sit with a box of truffles in one hand, an empty cup in the other, and derive the same pleasure simply by chewing, smacking, sucking, and then spitting as I do from swallowing.

I wonder if the gold-foiled candy holds a different flavor to stimulate my anxious palate. I pick one up and repeat the above process a second time. I'm not sure. Perhaps it's almond, but isn't that what amaretto is? I eat another red one—hmmm, still not sure—but I do know that I like them both equally well, so I unwrap another gold one, then another red one, and so on, and so on.

Before the end of the mitten party I had eaten thirty milk chocolate truffles. I still couldn't have said if they were the same or different; and I had yet to expose myself to trays of fudge and cookies downstairs on the center island in the kitchen. Between the truffles, trays of chocolate pastries, a plate of cream-filled somethings, frosted sugar cookies, and a quart of ice-cold skim milk because it's hard to imagine the one without the others, I had consumed between eight and ten thousand Calories.

Was I crazy hungry from not eating all day? *No.* Did I even miss supper? *No.* Why, then, did I do it? Obsessive-compulsive behavior, food addiction—I couldn't say for sure. What I do know is that it was a pattern of eating with me—not being able to stop.

One month later I found myself sitting in the galley of a sailboat en route to Miami from Bimini. I had given each of my two accompanying brothers-in-law Dramamine tablets I had brought along. Both of them had gotten violently ill on the crossing to Bimini the week before, although they had taken the medication prior to that as well. As for myself, I have never been seasick a day in my life and to impress upon them my natural-born seaworthiness, I ate breakfast. Since no one else wanted to eat, in the hopes of avoiding repeated episodes of projectile emesis, I had plenty to pick from.

"Are you sure you don't want any of these pancakes, Fred?" I ask brother-in-law number one. The bitter taste of partially digested hamburgers and baked beans spraying geyser-like from his mouth last week is too recent a memory. He declines. I slather butter on each pancake in a stack of three, drench everything in syrup, add blueberries, and then top everything off with half a pressurized can of whipped cream—phht, phhhhhhhht.

"You're nuts," says brother-in-law number two.

"Hey, I can't help it if you guys have pussy stomachs. It must be genetic." I laugh while shoveling a forkful of pancakes/whipped cream/blueberries into my mouth.

"Pass the sausage, please," I ask Jim between swallows.

After the pancake stack, a few eggs, and several greasy pork sausage links, I feel that I am ready to take my measure on the crossing. As a further emphasis, I savor a couple of stale cinnamon rolls which have been in a plastic wrapper all week, but they freshened up considerably in the microwave.

Halfway through the Bimini chop I'm feeling only just okay. The seas are rough, with eight- to twelve-foot rollers that lift and drop the boat, like a one-story elevator, on ten-second intervals. Up, there's the sky; down, there's the ocean; up and down, up and down, sky and ocean…sky, ocean…ocean, I forget, didn't I just see sky? Suddenly I'm dizzy. The ocean and sky are going around and around in addition to up and down. At the end of every down part, the bow of the vessel plows into the leading roller, sending a sheet of icy spray raining onto the deck, making it impossible to stay dry. I sit behind the bulkhead, in front of the stairs going down into the galley, so I can watch the horizon while being slightly shielded from the spray. I'm afraid that I may have overestimated my seaworthiness. I feel as though there is a balloon that is being inflated inside of my stomach. Uh-oh. I open my mouth and release a wet burp containing a few flecks of sausage. I feel better. Relieved, I swallow the sausage again, this time without my customary enjoyment. Jim bumps past me at that point and takes my picture on his way downstairs to visit the head.

Two weeks later I am sitting in front of my computer, watching a slide show from the picture CD that Jim sent me. The pictures change at one-and-a-half-second intervals. The turquoise blue of the Caribbean fills the screen—then a scenic island in the distance with a lighthouse and a solitary palm tree—then a fat man on a sailboat. For some small fraction of a second I don't recognize myself. I freeze the image. It is me. In the rest of the pictures, towards the end, I find one of a moonfaced, obese man sitting in a puddle of water. I remember the picture that Jim took of me after breakfast during the crossing. This is where I begin to change. It takes a long time. I am on mostly an Atkins-type diet for more than a year; eighteen months later I complete my first sprint-distance triathlon at a weight of 239 lb.

#

I weigh 215 lb. today, in the month of October, 2008, five years and some months after that seminal moment in which I saw myself for the first time as a fat man on a sailboat. I have changed emotionally. I have changed physically. I am not the person I once was.

I have a three-hundred-page message to share—a message that has coalesced from my years of medical practice, a lifetime of personal experience, insightful contributions from my beautiful wife, and intensive research in a quest to find answers to my questions of *how* and *why*—and if not to know the answer, then at least to understand the question. I know a way to becoming the person that you want to be. It has taken me several years, with the most dramatic change occurring these past few years. It doesn't have to take as long for you, and it starts right about now. As for me, true awareness began early one morning, seemingly no different than any other, in, of all places, the master bathroom.

"Honey," I yelled, softly, because it was early. I heard her stir and asked, "Where's the scale?"

"It's in the basement, under the stairs."

I stood in the toilet room, naked, looking at the twelve-inch tile underneath the mirror where our sleek, electronic, body-fat-calculating, BMI-measuring scale used to be, wondering, *what the hell?*

Having been married for more than twenty years, Sue could read my mind and so she added, "It was stressing me out, weighing myself all the time. I'm not weighing myself anymore—and you weigh yourself too much too!"

As she drifted back off to sleep, I admitted to myself that she had a point. I weighed myself a lot. Some days, when my wedding ring was tight, I weighed myself reluctantly because I knew that my weight would be up, and not by a few pounds either. Every morning as I'd sit on the toilet, taking care of the daily business, sliding my wedding ring up and down on my finger, I'd wonder— *hmm… will this be a good day or a bad day?* Naturally, the definition of a bad day was when my ring would be tight on a thick third finger. Usually I could correlate a tight-ring day with a deep-dish Meat Lover's pizza or a couple of baskets of chips and salsa the day before. I now know that these daily fluctuations were more related to fluid retention than an increase in fat mass; but, even back then, I don't think knowing that would have made the four-pound weight gain on a tight-ring day any easier.

I weighed myself after exercising, to calculate my water loss and nutritional needs, I would tell Sue, but I was mostly interested in seeing how much I'd lost, even though I knew that it was mostly fluid, only a tall glass of water short of re-manifestation. Some mornings I would weigh myself three or four times: before my shower, after my shower, after a significant bowel movement and sometimes twice in a row, because I didn't think the scale was functioning properly the first time.

Ten months passed without a scale in the bathroom. Although Sue hadn't weighed herself during that period of time, she had gone through three wardrobe changes, which triggered a sharp uptick in the number of well-dressed women in Northeastern Wisconsin due to the sudden influx of designer, brand-name clothing flooding the thrift shops in Green Bay and Door County.

I am not too familiar with women's sizes, and when hauling off bags of size eighteens to St. Vincent De Paul I thought *eighteen what?* Eighteen inches? I didn't think so—maybe eighteen *double* inches. I didn't think eighteen sounded so bad. I mean, after all, I was wearing size forty-four jeans. *Would that make me a women's twenty-two?* Even they were tight. A couple of months later I was carrying out size sixteens and fourteens, a few months after that I found myself donating leftovers of the above and a few baggy twelves. By this time, I was including stacks of my own clothes, having gradually diminished to the point where I was wearing a size seventeen neck instead of twenty, and a thirty-four waist. Thankfully, our shoe sizes remained the same, because all this weight loss was getting expensive.

Everywhere we went, friends and acquaintances remarked on how well Sue looked and they begged her to share her *secret* with them. I, myself, was the recipient of compliments and questions of how I did it; and, when I told them that it was due mainly to obsessive-compulsive exercise, there was a quick loss of interest.

I attained my first physical peak July 27, 2005, at age forty-four, about a year prior to my gradually dawning awareness. I had just completed a sprint triathlon in one hour and fourteen minutes, and my wife took a picture of me under the "Door County Triathlon" sign. As soon as I got home, I started eating frosted sugar cookies; then there was Thanksgiving and pumpkin Bombay cheesecake dessert and more sugar cookies; then there were Christmas parties, more cheesecake and really big frosted sugar cookies, chocolate-covered cherries, macaroons, and, well, you get the idea. My newfound washboard abs sank into oblivion and all my new clothes stayed on their hangers.

I surrendered control of my weight loss program to my wife in the fall of 2006. She had discovered *a way.*

Her method was based on common sense, exercise, and counting calories, which is how I started out; but then I began to make changes based upon my reading and research that dealt with the science of nutrition and weight loss. Time passed, and once again the questions came. How did you do it? What is your secret?

This time, it was different. I had an answer. The problem was I couldn't answer the question in a few minutes, or even a few hours. How could I just say that it was because we didn't eat as much and exercised more? That's what everyone says. It sounded empty, meaningless, and not very helpful. I couldn't say *it was through a personal journey of discovery that effected a transformational lifestyle change* because that would have been meaningless as well. I needed to do much more.

Sue is my inspiration. She started me on my way with a simple command. After a couple of years of near constant reading and making eye contact over the rim of half-moon magnifiers, she said one day, "Why don't you write a book or something?"

So I did. I have written about everything that I have found pertinent to weight loss, which just so happens to correlate directly with happiness and a healthy lifestyle. I am inviting you on this journey of discovery that I like to think of as a process of *enlightenment.*

As a practicing general surgeon, I have dealt with obesity both personally and professionally for many years and am no stranger to it. Four years ago, when I sat in front of a blank Word document for the first time to put my thoughts and feelings into words, I didn't think it would take so long. There were many times during the course of composition when it seemed as though I were light-years away from writing on weight loss, but I felt that it all mattered. It mattered to me, and so I thought it might matter to you as well.

The problem with most diet books is that they are rather sterile and full of meal plans telling you specifically what to eat and when to eat it.

For example:

Breakfast—hard-boiled egg, one half of a grapefruit, one slice whole wheat toast, lightly buttered (low-fat).

Lunch—one-half can of tuna on one slice whole wheat toast, one 6 oz. glass of skim milk, garden salad with low-fat dressing, apple.

Supper—one skinless cooked chicken breast on bed of black rice, five spears of asparagus, and four oz. of whatever.

For variety, there are different meal plans for different days of the week. Half of the book will be composed of recipes; sometimes pages will be filled with blanks to be filled in. The problem is that at the end of the meal plan, at the end of the diet—then what? Diets, as we think of them, change the way you naturally eat and so at the end of the diet *you tend to eat naturally* again. Even a maintenance plan is forced and unnatural to any given dieter in the sense that it is a plan. You can't plan all your meals for the rest of your life, or I suppose you could, but that would make you obsessive-compulsive and most people call that *crazy.*

My objective is to tell you what you need to know in order to precipitate a positive change in the course of your life. It's not so much changing how you eat as it is *changing how you think.* This is what I am calling the relativity diet *a diet theory of everything* (DTOE), which is in reference to the holy grail of physics: the theory of everything (TOE), or the grand unification theory. This long-sought-after theory will provide a melding of the classical physics of Einstein's theory of relativity with the modern physics of quantum theory. I call it relativity because the theory as I put it forth can mean different things for different people. It is all relative to their frame of reference. I also call it relativity because that means time, space and energy, which pretty much sums up what life is all about.

I consider *The Relativity Diet: A Diet Theory of Everything* to be the holy grail of weight loss in the sense that it works. It worked for me. It will work for you.

This will not be a quick read. How could it possibly be? In order for me to help you lose weight permanently and lead a healthier lifestyle, you require a certain knowledge and understanding. I need to touch you somewhere deep inside to flip an imaginary switch that will change you in such a way that anything becomes possible. Although this book is within the diet book genre, it is much more than that—it is a life-changing book. I will tell you what types of foods you should eat and why. You will need to pick from these types of foods those that you would *naturally* be interested in. You may need to expand your interests somewhat—we'll see. This will involve more work than peeling plastic wrappers off of expensive frozen TV dinners received in the mail from a mail-order diet plan; but think of how much money you'll save and, as time goes on, you will take ownership and responsibility of your daily diet. I will eventually share with you a commonsense approach to eating, caveats of exercise, and how to increase your metabolic rate and maximize fat metabolism. But, first we must learn the importance of *being happy.*

This will not be short, this will not be easy, but this will last a lifetime. If you believe, if you understand and comply, then six to twelve months after reading this you will possess an appropriate body weight, and eating an appropriately balanced diet will be as natural as breathing. This is not the book for you if your goal is to lose weight for a wedding six weeks away, although the middle section *will* get you there. This is the book for you if you are ready to empower yourself so that you may make a positive change in your life.

There will be times you will think *what in the hell has this to do with weight loss?* Please, have patience, open your mind, relax, and wonder—wonder of us, a quintessence of dust in a vast universe of space.

chapter three

Fat facts

A CCORDING TO THE NATIONAL Center for Health Statistics, which falls under the jurisdiction of the Centers for Disease Control and prevention (CDC), the prevalence of overweight and obese adults in the United States exceeds 66 percent. This represents a steady increase from the initial collection of data in the early sixties when the prevalence of overweight and obese adults was 44.8 percent. More recent data, from 2006, has demonstrated no statistically significant increase from the 2003–2004 data.[1] I suppose you could say that this leveling off is good news, but, given that the data also demonstrates an increase in the prevalence of overweight children and adolescents, one might argue that the plateau is only momentary. Data collected from the mid-sixties through 2004 for children, ages 6–11, demonstrates an increase in the prevalence of overweight from 4.2 to 18.8 percent and for adolescents, ages 12–19, an increase from 4.6 to 17.4 percent.[1]

Globesity

Sadly, this epidemic of overweight and obesity has progressed to such a point that it is almost normal to be overweight, in the sense that the majority of us are. The United States has one of the highest incidences of obesity among industrialized nations; however, obesity has now become a worldwide problem and is on a steady upwards trajectory. What had once been thought to be a problem limited to high-income countries is now expanding to low- and mid-income countries, where the incidence of obesity is rising dramatically. The World Health Organization (WHO) defines overweight as a BMI ≥ 25 and projects that 2.3 billion adults will be overweight by the year 2015. In 2005 the WHO estimated the worldwide prevalence of overweight adults at 1.6 billion and overweight children under the age of five at 20 million.[2]

This increase in overweight and obesity is obvious to those with thirty or more years of conscious memory, and it has become such a widespread problem today that our young people don't remember when it wasn't. Evidence of obesity is wherever people gather: at the mall, in church, *or on a school playground.* You cannot read a newspaper or open a magazine without being exposed to a new weight loss drug, surgical procedure, or promise of thinness by buying this or doing that. I remember a time when most people weren't overweight, and I have a memory that is as fresh today as it was thirty-five years ago.

Half of the asphalt playground lay in a long shadow cast by the three-story, brick school building. Since sum-

mer break was only two weeks away, it was warm enough in the early morning sun to be outside without jackets. Our physical education teacher, Mr. Peters, was one of the few lay teachers at my parochial school; I remember him as tall, lean and stern, and I was glad that I was not in his homeroom because I had the impression that I would not have lived up to his expectations. He had us all lined up against the eight-foot chain-link fence that kept the errant ball or child from escaping into the street. We were all boys, because Sister Beatrice had all the girls at the other end of the playground so as to avoid any improper happenings.

This was my least favorite class, that being physical education, and would remain so throughout all the years then stretching out before me. I drew some consolation in the fact that at least I wouldn't be the last one picked. I knew that would be Darrell. Darrell was the one fat kid in our class of twenty-six. He was no taller or shorter than most of us, but he was quite round, similar to my uncle Bob, who I strongly suspected was the Santa who came to our house on Christmas Eve because he only came over after Santa left, and they both had the smell of beer on their breaths.

I know that Darrell dreaded this part of the day as much as I did, because he always stood next to me, nervous and tense and sucking in his stomach so as to not appear so heavy. Sometimes our eyes would meet—an emotional connection of fear, both of us frightened at what embarrassment might lie before us over the next hour.

"Shaun," my team captain called indifferently. I trotted off to join seven or eight others.

"Darrell." The other team captain's voice as he called out his name may have been slightly less enthusiastic than the voice calling mine but if it was, I found no consolation in it.

The real stars of St. Mary's playground were called out in loud excited voices, accompanied by bursts of physicality like a pumping fist, a bouncing up and down on the balls of one's feet, or an ardent pointing towards the athletic star of the moment. "I'll take Mike" or "Tommy" or...insert name of thin, average-height, male child. Often this would be followed by an "all right!" or "yeah!" As the selections continued, there would become less and less excitement, until, towards the end, there remained only the champions of mediocrity and disappointment.

Although I was not as heavy as Darrell, I was no better an athlete. I suppose I just looked better, which allowed for my earlier selection. I couldn't run fast without tripping and I couldn't catch any sort of ball whatsoever. When I think back, I know that it was a function of my peripheral nervous system catching up to oversized arms and legs and an undiagnosed nearsightedness, but at the time it remained an unexplained and painful mystery.

I don't know what became of Darrell. For all I know, he could be reed thin today. What I do know is that thirty to forty years ago there was one Darrell in a class of twenty-six; now there are nearly five. Forty years ago, in elementary school, one would be graded on a scale of some sort; there would be winners and losers, and playground schoolteachers divided children into teams, one at a time, based on physical prowess. Now kids are graded as pass/fail and there are no losers, only winners, and playground schoolteachers divide up the children in a more sensitive manner. Does this make it any easier on the overweight and obese children? I think not. I suspect the other children see to that. The only positive outcome of the increase in overweight children is that each might not feel so alone; but, of course, that does not make it right or acceptable.

This is the slippery slope of obesity, where so many are overweight that it becomes almost normal and thereby acceptable to be overweight, because the majority of us are. In gross numbers, 66 percent of all US adults equals 133.6 million overweight or obese people. Of this number, 65.4 million, or 32.3 percent of all US adults, are obese.[3] In addition to the emotional cost of being overweight, there are also health-related costs, which translate into considerable economic costs as well.

Body mass index

The most common classification of body weight by which the overweight and obese are defined is the body mass index (BMI). The BMI is equal to body mass or weight, in kilograms, divided by height, in meters squared, and is easily derived from readily available tables of height and weight. The table is the same for both men and women. As an example, a six-foot individual (72 inches) who weighs 184 pounds would have a BMI of 25, which is considered overweight. The same individual with a body mass of 221 pounds would have a BMI of 30, which is considered obese.

Obesity Class	BMI (kg/m^2)
Underweight	< 18.5
Normal	18.5–24.9
Overweight	25.0–29.9
Obesity I	30.0–34.9
Obesity II	35.0–39.9
Extreme obesity III	> 40

Body Mass Index Table

To use the table, find the appropriate height in the left-hand column labeled Height. Move across to a given weight. The number at the top of the column is the BMI at that height and weight. Pounds have been rounded off.

BMI	Normal						Overweight					Obese										Extreme Obesity														
	19	20	21	22	23	24	25	26	27	28	29	30	31	32	33	34	35	36	37	38	39	40	41	42	43	44	45	46	47	48	49	50	51	52	53	54
Height (inches)												Body Weight (pounds)																								
58	91	96	100	105	110	115	119	124	129	134	138	143	148	153	158	162	167	172	177	181	186	191	196	201	205	210	215	220	224	229	234	239	244	248	253	258
59	94	99	104	109	114	119	124	128	133	138	143	148	153	158	163	168	173	178	183	188	193	198	203	208	212	217	222	227	232	237	242	247	252	257	262	267
60	97	102	107	112	118	123	128	133	138	143	148	153	158	163	168	174	179	184	189	194	199	204	209	215	220	225	230	235	240	245	250	255	261	266	271	276
61	100	106	111	116	122	127	132	137	143	148	153	158	164	169	174	180	185	190	195	201	206	211	217	222	227	232	238	243	248	254	259	264	269	275	280	285
62	104	109	115	120	126	131	136	142	147	153	158	164	169	175	180	186	191	196	202	207	213	218	224	229	235	240	246	251	256	262	267	273	278	284	289	295
63	107	113	118	124	130	135	141	146	152	158	163	169	175	180	186	191	197	203	208	214	220	225	231	237	242	248	254	259	265	270	278	282	287	293	299	304
64	110	116	122	128	134	140	145	151	157	163	169	174	180	186	192	197	204	209	215	221	227	232	238	244	250	256	262	267	273	279	285	291	296	302	308	314
65	114	120	126	132	138	144	150	156	162	168	174	180	186	192	198	204	210	216	222	228	234	240	246	252	258	264	270	276	282	288	294	300	306	312	318	324
66	118	124	130	136	142	148	155	161	167	173	179	186	192	198	204	210	216	223	229	235	241	247	253	260	266	272	278	284	291	297	303	309	315	322	328	334
67	121	127	134	140	146	153	159	166	172	178	185	191	198	204	211	217	223	230	236	242	249	255	261	268	274	280	287	293	299	306	312	319	325	331	338	344
68	125	131	138	144	151	158	164	171	177	184	190	197	203	210	216	223	230	236	243	249	256	262	269	276	282	289	295	302	308	315	322	328	335	341	348	354
69	128	135	142	149	155	162	169	176	182	189	196	203	209	216	223	230	236	243	250	257	263	270	277	284	291	297	304	311	318	324	331	338	345	351	358	365
70	132	139	146	153	160	167	174	181	188	195	202	209	216	222	229	236	243	250	257	264	271	278	285	292	299	306	313	320	327	334	341	348	355	362	369	376
71	136	143	150	157	165	172	179	186	193	200	208	215	222	229	236	243	250	257	265	272	279	286	293	301	308	315	322	329	338	343	351	358	365	372	379	386
72	140	147	154	162	169	177	184	191	199	206	213	221	228	235	242	250	258	265	272	279	287	294	302	309	316	324	331	338	346	353	361	368	375	383	390	397
73	144	151	159	166	174	182	189	197	204	212	219	227	235	242	250	257	265	272	280	288	295	302	310	318	325	333	340	348	355	363	371	378	386	393	401	408
74	148	155	163	171	179	186	194	202	210	218	225	233	241	249	256	264	272	280	287	295	303	311	319	326	334	342	350	358	365	373	381	389	396	404	412	420
75	152	160	168	176	184	192	200	208	216	224	232	240	248	256	264	272	279	287	295	303	311	319	327	335	343	351	359	367	375	383	391	399	407	415	423	431
76	156	164	172	180	189	197	205	213	221	230	238	246	254	263	271	279	287	295	304	312	320	328	336	344	353	361	369	377	385	394	402	410	418	426	435	443

Source: Adapted from *Clinical Guidelines on the Identification, Evaluation, and Treatment of Overweight and Obesity in Adults: The Evidence Report.*

The cost of obesity

According to the National Heart, Lung, and Blood Institute (NHLBI), a branch of the National Institutes of Health, the total cost attributed to obesity amounted to 99.2 billion dollars in 1995. Of this, 51.6 billion represented the direct medical costs of obesity, and indirect costs of 47.6 billion represented lost economic output due to mortality (death) and morbidity (illness).[4] Allowing for inflation and an increase in prevalence of ten percent, the total economic cost in 2008 dollars is around 148 billion dollars a year.

As if the economic costs were not sobering enough, consider the burden of the obese in regard to illness and death or, as we say in medicine, morbidity and mortality. Morbid (extreme) obesity is the definition reserved for those unfortunate enough to be in possession of a BMI of greater than 40. I think that a more appropriate term would be *mortal obesity* because that implies death rather than illness, and it is nearly a given that the morbidly obese will die prematurely of a cause relating to their obesity. The medical literature clearly shows that being overweight or obese substantially increases the risk of morbidity from the following: hypertension; dyslipidemia (high cholesterol); type 2 diabetes; coronary heart disease; stroke; gallbladder disease; osteoarthritis, sleep apnea and respiratory problems; and endometrial, breast, prostate, and colon cancers.[5]

Apart from the economic and health-related costs, which are staggering by themselves, are the very significant emotional costs that all overweight and obese people bear to some extent. Whether obesity is the result of or the cause of emotional distress is of no matter—in

either case it needs to be addressed; however, it may be
that some emotional issues will need to be addressed
in order for significant and long-lasting weight loss to
occur.

Obesity and inflammation

I have a personal interest in the relationship between
obesity and inflammation because I contracted a serious,
uncommon heart condition in the spring of 2001 that
was of an inflammatory nature. The problem was with
my pericardium, which is a sac that surrounds the heart.
In medicine there is a term, *idiopathic,* which means that
we do not have a clue as to the cause of some illness or
condition. Well, I had a severe case of idiopathic, chronic
relapsing pericarditis, which meant that my pericardium
was inflamed. It is like someone hit it with a hammer, in
the sense that when you hit your thumb with a hammer
or get it stuck in a door, it gets all swollen and black and
blue and throbs with each beat of your heart—that's
what my pericardium was like. My cardiologist thought
that it may have been virus induced. Sue thought that it
was from the bacterial counts in the bay of Sturgeon Bay
that I was so fond of swimming in. My anesthesiologist
friend, Brutus, thought it was from holding my breath
too long while free-diving. Now, years later, during my
research on obesity, I wondered if it could have been
related to my BMI of 39.

Inflammation plays a vital role in the body's defenses.
Everyone has experienced the inflammatory process
firsthand at some point in their lives. Simply recall an
adverse encounter with a kitchen knife, a fall from your
bike, a twisted ankle; or, in the unlikely event that you
have been trauma-free your entire life and you wish to

experience the inflammatory response unequivocally, do this: rest your left thumb on a firm surface, like a cement floor or piece of wood, and with a full-sized hammer strike the nail bed squarely with the force equivalent to that of driving a picture nail into a two-by-four stud.* This shouldn't break anything, and will give a nice example of heat, redness, swelling, and pain, which just so happen to be the hallmarks of inflammation.

The primary impetus for the inflammatory response is tissue injury, with the leakage of plasma and blood cells into the soft tissues. The result is a cascade of events involving the release of chemical mediators from the tissues and circulating cells. These mediators are responsible for the pain and swelling, over and above that due to the stimulation of regional pain fibers and tissue edema (swelling) from the direct injury itself.

The inflammatory process is a vital part of the immune system and, as such, defects in the immune system lie at the root of many systemic illnesses: auto-immune disorders such as lupus, rheumatoid arthritis and inflammatory bowel disease; diabetes; vascular disease; and malignancy are all examples. In recent years, research has shown that one of the defects of the immune system is related to obesity.

Obesity is associated with an elevation in the tissue and blood level concentrations of the chemical mediators of the inflammatory response. It seems that the mature fat cell, which is also called an adipocyte, has the capacity to synthesize and secrete these very same mediators of inflammation. With an increase in fat cells,

---

*   Obviously, I am suggesting this contextually, not literally; and if you
    still elect to proceed with said demonstration—it is at your own peril.

particularly in the case of visceral obesity (fat inside the abdomen), there are increased levels of these mediators circulating in the bloodstream with the net effect being a *pro-inflammatory* state. The fat cells, comprising the white adipose tissue, are not an inert mass that merely expands or shrinks relative to what we eat or don't eat. The white adipose tissue is more like a gland, and when the "gland" is bigger it is more active, and when it becomes smaller it is less active. If there is an increase in the white adipose tissue—*bigger gland*—then there are elevated levels of the chemical mediators of inflammation and this leads to a pro-inflammatory state, which represents a low-grade, chronic inflammatory condition that is a systemic process, with systemic effects on parts of the body far removed from the fat deposits. If there is a decrease in the white adipose tissue—*smaller gland*—then the levels of chemical mediators will fall with a lessening of the pro-inflammatory state.

An example of a harmful effect of the pro-inflammatory state would be the white blood cells that are traveling throughout the body via the blood vessels. Due to the elevated levels of the chemical mediators of inflammation, the white blood cells are also in a pro-inflammatory state and are involved in plaque buildup in the arterial vessels, which contributes to impaired circulation of blood. The combined effect of the obesity-related changes of this chronic inflammatory state contributes to the development of insulin resistance and diabetes, cardiovascular disease (CVD), stroke, and certain types of cancer. Encouragingly, the research has also demonstrated that the pro-inflammatory state is reversible with weight loss.[6,7,8]

Obesity and the metabolic syndrome

The chronic inflammatory state associated with obesity correlates with a collection of metabolic and physiologic abnormalities collectively known as the metabolic syndrome. Although this was first suggested in the twenties, it was not until the 1980s that it began receiving more attention. International and national expert groups, such as the WHO, International Diabetes Foundation, and the National Cholesterol Education Program, have proposed similar definitions, of which the primary components of the syndrome are insulin resistance, glucose intolerance, central obesity, increased levels of circulating triglycerides (fat), decreased levels of good cholesterol, and hypertension. Impaired glucose tolerance is an intermediate stage in the natural history of type 2 diabetes and is highly predictive of diabetes and cardiovascular disease.

The prevalence of the metabolic syndrome has been shown to be increasing dramatically throughout the world, parallel to the rising incidence of obesity. This increase has also been demonstrated in children, again demonstrating a direct correlation with obesity. As the metabolic syndrome is a precursor to diabetes, type 2 diabetes is no longer a disease of primarily adults. The CDC estimates that one in three newborns of the twenty-first century will eventually develop diabetes during the course of their lifetime.[7,9]

Medical diseases associated with obesity

Clearly, obesity is not a desirable condition, other than maybe for the purpose of sumo wrestling, and it can be definitively linked to significant medical illness and death via associations with the chronic inflammatory state and the metabolic syndrome. A major study was published in the *Journal of the American Medical Association*[10] in November of 2007, which analyzed data from national surveys compiled by the National Center for Health Statistics and US vital statistics. The surveys represented cross-sectional samples of the US population and were collected in a standardized fashion from 36,859 people, with a length of follow-up ranging up to as long as twenty-nine years.

Deaths were grouped into three major categories: cardiovascular disease, cancer, and all other causes (non-cancer, non-CVD). The results obtained identified excess deaths related to obesity and the cancers considered to be obesity related, which are listed below. Interestingly, for non-cancer, non-CVD mortality, underweight was associated with a significant number of excess deaths and overweight with a significant *negative* number of excess deaths (fewer people died), suggesting a protective effect of being overweight (not obese) in the non-cancer, non-CVD deaths. However, when kidney disease and diabetes were separated out from the other non-cancer, non-CVD deaths, overweight *was* associated with an increased mortality.

Obesity-related cancers

Colon
Breast
Esophageal
Uterine
Ovarian
Kidney
Pancreatic

Excess Deaths in the United States in 2004 Associated with a BMI > 30 (Obese)	
Cardiovascular Disease	112,159
Cancer	15,252
Non-cancer, non-CVD	35,594
Total	163,005

In reviewing the medical literature, it is clear that the most significant risk of morbidity and mortality, secondary to obesity, is CVD. The second most significant risk of morbidity and mortality, secondary to overweight and obesity, is the diabetes and kidney disease fraction of the non-cancer and non-CVD population. The excess deaths secondary to cancer in the obese population, although not as impressive as the first two, is not insignificant.

The metabolic syndrome and the pro-inflammatory state of obesity play a key role in the morbidity and mortality of the overweight and obese, with the final common pathway being the development of diabetes, kidney disease, CVD, cancer, and, ultimately, premature death if the obesity goes unchecked.[11]

All of the above material is very technical information and may be somewhat confusing to the lay reader. I presented it because although it represents one of the more conservative estimates of the impact of obesity, it represents the data in a very rigorous and unbiased fashion. The bottom line in all of this is that obesity is a systemic process. The obese patient doesn't get only diabetes, or only heart disease, or only kidney disease or only an elevated risk of cancer—the obese patient gets a little of everything, to varying degrees. Whereas one obese patient might have primarily coronary artery

disease and a whiff of diabetes requiring only oral medication, another obese patient may be insulin dependent
and suffering from kidney disease while having only
mild coronary artery disease. Obesity represents a
spectrum of illness and of death, which is treatable and
reversible with weight loss. *So let's get busy.*

chapter four

Fat classification & body types

T HE CLASSIFICATION OF OVERWEIGHT and obesity, and body type is much more complex than the application of the BMI table. A "normal" BMI may not be appropriate for an individual who has a large frame or muscular build; therefore, we will discuss various classification systems, some of more utility than others.

Fat morphology

Morphology is defined as the structure and form of an organism, excluding its function; therefore, when I say "fat morphology" I am referring to the structure and form of the fat of an organism, namely the Homo sapiens. A common classification of body type that may sound familiar is ectomorphic (thin), like Kevin Bacon; mesomorphic (muscular), like Arnold Schwarzenegger or Russell Crowe; and endomorphic (fat), like the late Chris Farley. I think that it is easier to assign these categories to men, as their musculature is more on display, as opposed to the female physique. In an attempt at gender equality I will go out on a limb and label the female ecto-, meso-, and endomorph body types as Angelina Jolie, Kirstie Alley, and Kirstie Alley. Ms. Alley is an example of a mesomorph in the occasional disguise of an endomorph—I think she is beautiful in both cases. The ecto-, meso-, and endomorph classification is a poor one in the sense that any endomorph could be either a fat ectomorph or a fat mesomorph—it's hard to say under all that fat. The endomorph doesn't know if he or she should say *actually, I'm quite muscular under all this fat* or *actually, I'm really very thin underneath my fat.*

A more objective classification is one of frame size, which is related to skeletal structure, and for which standardized anthropometric tables exist. If you must assign yourself a body frame size, don't automatically think that you are "big boned," or have a large frame, just because you weigh a lot. This makes it easy to rationalize something to the effect—*I can eat more, like that two-pound piece of carrot cake, because I'm big boned.* You may not be as *big* as you think you are. I suggest using the supplied tables for an accurate frame size assignment. The primary utility of the body frame size is to identify those people who may be incorrectly classified as *overweight*, based on their BMI, because of a *medium* or *large* body frame.

How to calculate your body frame size

Standardized anthropometric tables of elbow breadth and wrist circumference are an easy way to assign a specific body type.

Elbow breadth measurement

Of the two measurements, the elbow breadth is perhaps more technically challenging. The tables listed below include the elbow breadth measurements for a medium-sized frame, relative to height, for both male and female. If your elbow breadth measurement is less than that of a medium frame, then you are considered to have a small frame; conversely, if your elbow breadth measurement is greater than the medium-sized frame, then you are considered to have a large frame.

To perform this measurement, extend your arm straight out in front with the palm facing upwards and then flex your arm at the elbow to 90 degrees so that your palm is facing you. This position allows you to measure the width of the ulnar bone which forms the "point" of the elbow, except that now it isn't really a point, but rather a transverse length. Pinch the narrowest part of the elbow (ulnar bone) in this flexed position and measure this distance, which represents the elbow breadth. Make sure that you do not measure the width of the humerus, which is further back.

Male elbow breadth measurement
for medium frame

Height (ft.–in.)	Elbow Breadth (in.)
5′ 2″–5′ 3″	2½″–2⅞″
5′ 4″–5′ 7″	2⅝″–2⅞″
5′ 8″–5′ 11″	2¾″–3″
6′ 0″–6′ 3″	2¾″–3⅛″
6′ 4″–6′ 7″	2⅞″–3¼″

Female elbow breadth measurement
for medium frame

Height (ft.–in.)	Elbow Breadth (in.)
4′ 10″–4′ 11″	2¼″–2½″
5′ 0″–5′ 3″	2¼″–2½″
5′ 4″–5′ 7″	2⅜″–2⅝″
5′ 8″–5′ 11″	2⅜″–2⅝″
6′ 0″–6′ 4″	2½″–2¾″

Wrist measurement

This is relatively easier to accomplish than the elbow breadth but it does not provide quite the range of the former. It is as simple as measuring the circumference of your wrist with a flexible tape measure.

Male Wrist Measurements
(Height > 5′ 5″)

Frame	Wrist
Small	5½″–6½″
Medium	6½″–7½″
Large	> 7½″

Female Wrist Measurements

Frame	Height < 5′ 2″	Height 5′ 2″–5′ 5″	Height > 5′ 5″
Small	< 5½″	< 6″	< 6¼″
Medium	5½″–5¾″	6″–6¼″	6¼″–6½″
Large	> 5¾″	> 6¼″	> 6½″

I have to admit that my own wrist measurement is a pedestrian 7¼ inches and my elbow breadth a mere 2½ inches, which at 6 feet 3 inches puts me comfortably in the medium category when all these years I thought that I had the large frame of an NFL-caliber lineman.

Body fat patterning

A more descriptive classification of the morphology of fat pertains to the manner in which one gains weight, referred to as *body fat patterning*. A gross simplification would be that you either gain weight like a boy, or that you gain weight like a girl. The correct terminology is android obesity (apple shape) and gynoid obesity (pear shape). I will take the liberty of coining a third term, hermaphroid obesity, which may be thought of as being in the middle, between the two extremes of android and gynoid obesity; having features of both.

Because of the morbidity and mortality associated with obesity, it is viewed as a net negative by those in the medical profession excepting perhaps the bariatric surgeon, who derives his or her livelihood from the surgical treatment of the disease. While non-surgical physicians struggle with managing the challenging medical problems associated with the obese patient, surgical physicians, as am I, struggle with operating on and around the fat of the obese patient. Operating on the obese patient is technically more difficult due to the thickness of the abdominal wall and the large amount of fatty tissue surrounding the organs in the obese patient. The operations in obese people take longer, and most significantly, there is a higher risk of anesthetic, cardiopulmonary, and wound-healing complications.

I have not met a non-bariatric surgeon who didn't share my sentiment, and, given the prevalence of overweight and obesity, I see this on a daily basis, more often than not. If I were given a choice, however, of door number one, behind which stands an obese male, and door number two, behind which stands an obese female, I'll take door number two every time—the reason being the general differences in body fat patterning between men and women.

Performing an appendectomy on an obese man and an obese woman of an equivalent BMI provides a striking illustration of the different body fat patterns. Simply put, I find that the woman is fat on the outside but skinny, relatively, on the inside; whereas, the man is skinny, relatively, on the outside, but fat on the inside.

When I incise the soft belly of an obese female with my six inches of cold steel—*pet name for scalpel that I picked up in medical school from Dr. Swanson*—I'll easily cut through several inches of glistening, whitish-yellow fat before encountering the muscular layer of the abdomen, but at least when I open the belly it's easier to find the appendix. Conversely, when I incise the obese belly of a male, it is hard, rather than soft, because all the fat is on the inside, pushing out against the muscular layer. I may find only an inch or two of subcutaneous fat, but when I open the peritoneum (the lining of the abdominal cavity) the only thing I see is fat, everywhere. First I encounter the greater omentum, which is a fatty apron hanging down from the bottom of the stomach. This covers the internal organs in a thick, heavy blanket of fat. Then there is the investing fat that swallows up the intestines, especially the colon, which is what I am interested in ninety percent of the time anyway. It is, relatively speaking, the complete reverse of the obese female, and this is the simple, gross difference between android (male) and gynoid (female) obesity.

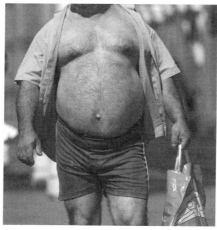

© Geronimo / Fotolia

Android obesity

Android obesity, commonly described as an "apple" shape, is more prevalent in men. It is also referred to as *central* or *visceral* obesity because of the increase in fat deposition in the abdominal area, specifically the visceral fat which surrounds the intestines, solid organs, and blood vessels. We all know people like this. Perhaps we are one of "those" people.

My uncle Bob, for instance, is a good example. For the past forty years he has looked pretty much the same: a pregnant belly having a convex slope from the base of his short, thick neck down to stork-thin legs with sagging flat buttocks. It seems as though, when he walks, he has to lean slightly back in order to counteract the weight of his overhanging belly, or else be pulled forward, perpetually off balance by the warped center of gravity of his abdominal girth.

One of the few nice things about visceral fat is that it is metabolically active and the fat mass will decrease dramatically with weight loss. Because of its central location, waist circumference is a more accurate assessment of visceral fat than the BMI, as the waist measurement differentiates central obesity from peripheral obesity, which we will discuss next. There are no standardized tables as with the BMI, but a general rule is—if the umbilical waist circumference is greater than the hip circumference, measured at the greatest girth of the buttocks (i.e., *your stomach is bigger than your butt*), then significant central obesity exists, along with the attendant health risks.

Sit-ups, antigravity boots, and vibrating machines will not make central obesity go away, unless the increased energy expenditure from doing the sit-ups, hanging upside down, or flipping the vibrating machine switch allows for a net caloric loss at the end of the day, which is exceedingly unlikely for the simple reason that the first two will more likely precipitate a strangulated hernia or stroke, and the third endeavor of flip switching and passive jiggling doesn't require that much energy. Clearly, the idea of dedicated abdominal exercises to decrease abdominal fat is somewhat intuitive, but they won't give you a six-pack unless you lose weight, thereby decreasing your body fat percentage. Everyone has a six-pack under their fat envelope. Even my 80-year-old cadaver in medical school had six-pack abs that would have been the envy of the beach—of course, this wasn't obvious until I dissected away a thick rind of subcutaneous tissue.

My consistent recommendation is that the primary management of waist circumference is dietary modification (caloric restriction). Exercise alone is also effective, but—a big butt, you might say—*only* if the net caloric balance is negative. The *easiest* way to decrease the abdominal girth is with dietary restriction. Four to six hours of exercise a week at a low to moderate level of activity would naturally accentuate that, as well as provide the cardiovascular benefit of aerobic exercise, and the musculoskeletal benefit of resistance training.

Gynoid obesity

If there were a *fat morphology scale* of one to ten, with android obesity having a value of one, then at the other end of the spectrum would be gynoid obesity, with a value of ten. Few people are at either extreme, just like anything else, and most fall somewhere in between. Gynoid obesity is more typical in females, and is also referred to as *peripheral obesity,* in which there is a preference for fat deposition in the hips and gluteal regions, accounting for a "pear" shape. Unfortunately, this fat is not as metabolically active as visceral fat and is generally the last place that fat stores are mobilized from. Peripheral

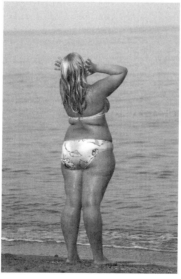

© Petro Feketa / Fotolia

obesity implies excess fat outside of the peritoneal cavity, as opposed to central obesity. Obviously, there is some degree of visceral obesity with all obese individuals, but in one with a gynoid-type body fat pattern there is a preponderance of peripheral obesity, as opposed to the visceral obesity of the android-type body fat pattern.

The most extreme—really far out on the very end of the bell curve extreme—case of gynoid obesity I have ever seen was a sixty-five-year-old, diabetic, hypertensive, arterial plaque–encrusted lady named Agnes, who was as good an example of the metabolic syndrome as you'll ever find. I can use her real name now because she's deceased; deceased from complications of morbid obesity, despite heroic efforts to make a difference with my six inches of cold steel.

The first time Agnes wheeled a well-worn walker with hand brakes into my office was because of her legs. At 58 inches and 209 pounds, her BMI of 43 qualified her as morbidly obese. Even if she were assigned a "credit" of two inches for the osteoporotic wedge compression fractures of her thoracic spine resulting in a marked dorsal kyphosis (stooped shoulders), her BMI would still be 41, comfortably within the morbidly obese category. Agnes suffered from a laundry list of medical problems, but her chief complaint that day was venous stasis disease.

Venous stasis disease is a common affliction of the obese, and Agnes was no exception. This is a problem, compounded by obesity, heart disease, and poor circulation, where there is impaired venous flow of the blood back to the heart from the legs. The lower legs become chronically swollen, and over time the skin turns brownish and shiny; the tissue develops a woody texture, and in the advanced stages ulcers develop. Agnes had big ulcers.

A common treatment for the ulcers is the application of a medicated-paste wrap called an Unna boot. From across the room, after one look at her ankles beneath the hem of her skirt, I could see that Agnes needed one on each leg. I examined her in the chair because I didn't want to make her move to the exam table, which would have involved the walker, additional staff, and six more tall inches of vertical height.

"Good morning, Agnes." I sat on the low stool that is in each of my exam rooms and wheeled over to assess the extent of her venous stasis disease. I primly lifted the hem of her skirt and saw that there were a couple of ulcers the size of silver dollars (*1924 Liberty head*), fairly shallow and not infected, just above the skinniest part of the ankle. I raised the faded calico print higher to get an idea of the proximal extent of her disease and saw that the brownish skin pigmentation changes extended to her—pannus? I realized that I couldn't see Agnes's knees because they were covered by a woody, discolored over-hanging belly of fat. When she stood up, her venous-static pannus hung down to her mid-shin level, a few inches above the hem of her skirt, which seemed to have been strategically hemmed at a level precisely of the length to tastefully cover her pendulant pannus. In order to apply the Unna boot, I had to have my nurse hold Agnes's pannus up and out of the way so that I could apply the wrap to just below the knee, if you could call it that; the knee being more like a couple of transverse wrinkles some-where in the middle of a thick, slightly tapering leg.

After three bilateral Unna boot applications, one week apart, I found Agnes's abdominal ulcer—and only then because of the note from her primary care physi-cian paper-clipped to the front of her chart: "please comment on Agnes's abdominal ulcer." So after the bilateral Unna boot applications, in the fourth week of our acquaintance, my nurse, Tree, and I muscled Agnes onto the electrified exam chair, from which I could convert her to a relative position of recumbency with foot pedals. I covered her legs with a paper drape and folded up her dress, which I thought would be more expedient than pulling it down. Tree and I looked, expectantly, at her abdomen. "Do you see any ulcer, Tree?"

"No."

"Help me lift this up," I said, and picked up my side of the pannus. Tree picked up her side and we flipped it up and onto Agnes's chest. A moist, fragrant, yeasty smell filled the room. I imagined twirling bacterial flagella and protoplasmic movements of unicellular organisms engaged in frenetic attempts to escape the harsh light and coldness of day.

"Ah, there it is," I said. Tree nodded in agreement, not wanting to open her mouth. She buried her nose in the sleeve of her blouse and sniffed cautious shallow breaths.

The ulcer was right in the middle of the skinfold of the undersurface of the pannus—the moist part. The skin-on-skin contact area was reddened and coated with curdled, whitish-yellow smegma, more commonly found on a fresh-born baby, or under the foreskin of an uncircumcised penis. The ulcer involved an oblong three inches of the skin crease, more above it than below. As I studied it, wondering what product I could possibly use to treat the ulcer, an idea germinated in the recesses of my right frontal lobe and rapidly intumesced to fruition, like a time-lapse film clip of a mammoth sunflower plant sprouting from seed to full grown in ten seconds.

"Tree," I said, reaching for Agnes's pedunculated pan-nus. "Pick the pannus up and hold it at ninety degrees, like this." I suspended the pannus in midair over Agnes's midsection, which was a good thing, because she was getting short of breath from the weight of her stomach on her chest.

It was as I thought. With Tree holding the pannus straight up I could easily approximate the normal skin beneath the ulcer, *below the pannus*, with the normal skin *above the pannus*. The majority of the fat in Agnes's pannus resided in its dependent portion. It was like she had an oversized football of fat, contained within a sub-cutaneous sac, and when I pinched the layers of the sac together with my hands just above the abdominal wall, but below the "football," my hands were separated by only a couple of inches.

I would cut out the ulcer, and Agnes's pannus along with it. She wouldn't have a belly that you could bounce a quarter off of, but at least it wouldn't be hanging down past her knees.

Most of my surgical cases are not memorable; the few that are, more often than not, are disturbing memo-ries rather than pleasant ones. Agnes was a little of both. It was an afternoon case, and by the time I got to the operating room she was already asleep on a table that I couldn't see because of her fat spilling over the sides. It was almost like she was levitating in midair, with her arms out and feet together in a horizontal crucifixion pose. What seemed like such a wonderful idea in my office a few days earlier didn't seem quite so wonderful anymore.

The anesthesiologist, Brutus, who knows me quite well, said, "You know, it's not too late to change your mind—not until you make that first cut." He smiled, knowing that I was thinking that very same thing.

"Hey, it's only skin and fat, right?" I left the room to scrub. I had in my mind an imagined sequence of events of how I wanted the case to go. It's kind of like a fantasy—where the most desirable course of each step of a procedure is the outcome—very little bleeding, no surprises, fast pace, everyone's amazed at your operative skill, etc. I do this mental imagery with most major operations. Sometimes the operation turns out like my fantasy, sometimes it does not.

Half an hour later I was somewhere definitely remote from my fantasy. The upper and lower edges of the healthy skin edges that were two inches apart in my office were more than twelve inches apart. The upper flap was three inches thicker than the lower one. I held the freshly amputated, forty-pound pannus in my arms. The space it had occupied, until just recently, was a gaping, fish-mouth abyss stretching from one side of the operating room table to the other. The widely separated precipices of flesh were like the two sides of a canyon, one taller than the other, the effect of which lent the disconcerting sense that I had cut Agnes in half; like a magician with a jagged-tooth tree saw, except that there was no lovely assistant hidden by a box. There was only Agnes. There was no box, and I certainly was no magician.

The only sounds in the room were the sonorous hiss of the mechanical lung and the electronic blips of the heart monitor. Not only was I far removed from my fantasy, not one person in that room had ever been in this particular place before, either.

"Holy shit! I think I cut her in half." The room erupted in nervous laughter. "It's only skin and fat," I reminded mostly myself.

This case wasn't difficult; it just looked that way. It was only different. In surgery, at least with big cases, there are many steps between the first and the final one; sometimes you can't imagine the final step until you whittle away at some of the in-between ones first.

One and a half hours from the time of the skin incision, I placed the last staple, approximating the last bit of skin of what now looked like a smiley-face incision. The end result was quite satisfying. I felt like a magician.

Agnes no longer had a pannus or a skin ulcer. She had instantly lost forty pounds. The memory of me lifting up the bloody pannus and shouting "specimen" before dropping it ceremoniously into the thirty-two gallon garbage pail would periodically be relived, years later, at the occasional operating room social function.

Agnes was the first and the last abdominoplasty patient I ever did—the last, not because I wasn't a plastic surgeon, but because I have never seen a patient since with such a degree of peripheral obesity in such a convenient configuration.

Android and gynoid body fat distribution are two extremes of a spectrum, with my uncle Bob on one end and Agnes on the other. Not all men have the android body fat pattern and not all women have the gynoid distribution. In fact, some women have an android distribution and some men have a gynoid distribution.

Hermaphroid obesity

This specific subpopulation of overweight and obese people consists of those that I refer to as *hermaphroditically* (not a real word, but it fits) obese. They have equal parts of both android and gynoid body fat patterning. Although common, given the prevalence of obesity these days, it is more common to trend one way or the other.

This is where I live—and I am almost exactly, if not exactly, in the middle. My weight gain is perfectly symmetrical. When I consume ten thousand Calories on Thanksgiving Day and the days before and after (you will see that I am telling you the truth) it seems as though my "skin envelope" expands uniformly, like the universe after the Big Bang. My face gets a little rounder, my pants tighter, my neckties shorter, my ring snugger, and my shoes smaller. I have to use one of those elastic button expanders for my shirt collar when I wear a tie so that my face doesn't turn blue. I have to sit down sideways at the movie theater because my butt doesn't fit between the armrests if I try to sit straight down. At this stage of obesity, if I sit down in a lawn chair to eat my two gallon bag of kettle corn, like during the 4th of July fireworks display, when I stand up the chair will stick to my ass because the plastic-topped aluminum tube armrests are wrapped around my hips as tenaciously as an adolescent's arms during a slow dance.

The skinny-fat person

It is also possible to have a significant amount of visceral fat and a low amount of peripheral fat. In effect, one could be *fat on the inside* but *skinny on the outside*. Because of the elevated amount of visceral fat, the skinny-fat person would have an increased probability of falling prey to the metabolic syndrome and its attendant risks of diabetes, cardiovascular heart disease, stroke, and hypertension, which may not be suspected because of a normal or only slightly elevated BMI. The skinny-fat person is described in the lay literature[12,13] as a person who has lost weight primarily by significant caloric restriction and a paucity of exercise. A combination of cardiovascular and resis-

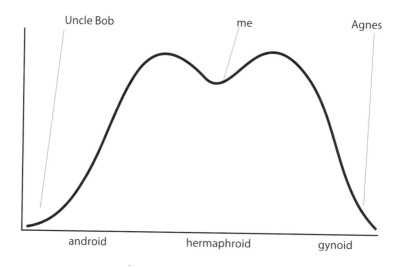

tance training is key in avoiding this and will be discussed in detail in the final section of the book.

A completely different classification

The BMI is a helpful classification of the overweight and obese for health-care providers because of its curvilinear relationship with the morbidity and mortality of the risk factors associated with obesity. I have in mind, however, a more simple classification that everyone fits neatly into—it is a very pragmatic one.

I checked my BMI recently and it was 29.3, which is what I got when I punched in my height on the scale in the men's locker room at our YMCA. That is a whisker under "obese—high health risk." The strange thing is that I am in great shape. I had just finished swimming 2,500 yards, and the elderly, blue-haired lady in the lane next to me told me how nice I looked. I can bench-press my wife several times. I can see my toes without bending over. So the BMI doesn't help my self-esteem very much. But apart from all that, apart from endomorph and

ectomorph and android and gynoid body fat distribu-
tions, there are basically two classes of overweight and
obese people. It's simple, really—there are those who
are trying to lose weight, and those who are not.

Those who are trying to lose weight

Of all the overweight and obese people trying to lose
weight, there are those who do and there are those who
do not. There are many, such as myself, who manage to
lose weight and a little while later find themselves in
the awkward position of having to lose it all over again
because they regained the weight shortly after they lost
it the first time. All of these people trying to lose weight
aren't trying because it's their hobby, although it seems
that way most of the time; they are trying because they
hate being fat. They don't like their shape; the tight
clothes; or perceived glances, smirks and whatever else,
imagined or otherwise, when out in public. This is the
street I used to live on.

Those who are losing weight are either doing it the
wrong way or the right way. The primary difference
between these is a matter of balance. Wrong-way dieters gain all their weight back over a relatively short
course of time, sometimes including a rebound gain of
additional weight. We all know people like this. One day
they're fat, the next day they're skinny, the following
day they're fat again—maybe we are even one of those
people.

Right-way dieters gradually lose weight over the
course of several months to a year or more. There is a
seismic change in their lives and outlook that translates
into lifestyle and behavioral modifications, which allows
their transformation from an endomorphic existence to

a mesomorphic or ectomorphic one. This is me now. This can be you.

Those who are not losing weight try *everything,* and nothing works. I hear this all the time from my patients. They'll tell me how much they've cut back on their eating, or decreased their fat intake, or increased their activity—all to no avail. There may be, however, a semblance of truth to this common complaint for a number of reasons. One cause of a failure to lose weight may be a drop in the metabolic rate—with a caloric restriction your metabolic rate drops; therefore, so do your daily energy requirements (calories), the net effect very possibly being no net change in weight because the reduction in caloric intake is offset by the energy savings of the decreased metabolic rate. This slowing of the metabolic rate is accentuated by skipping meals (fasting response), which causes your body to *conserve* energy, in anticipation of starving.

A second possible cause of a failure to lose weight may be the relative state of hydration—in the first few weeks of weight loss a larger proportion of the loss represents the water weight, contained in the body's energy stores, that is initially metabolized. The dieter may therefore rapidly gain back his or her weight after a few weeks of dieting, if straying off the diet for a day. The end result may be discouragement and abandonment of any attempt at caloric restriction. It is important to realize that daily weight change is more a reflection of the relative state of hydration, which is variable from day to day, rather than a reflection of any significant change in fat mass.

The longer you diet—and by that I mean several weeks to months—the more proportionate loss of fat there is. Water makes up about 70 percent of the weight lost over the first week of caloric restriction. In the second to fourth weeks of dieting, body fat loss increases from 25 percent to 70 percent, and by the fourth week of weight loss body fat accounts for 85 percent of weight loss.[14]

Finally, there are those trapped for several years, if not a lifetime, in the harsh sine wave of cyclical obesity, which may be more harmful than simply remaining *obesely* stable because of the repeated cardiac stresses of going from fat to thin over and over. I went through five cycles in fifteen years, losing weight, getting thinner, and then regaining weight, getting fatter again, and a little while later, thinner, then fatter, and so on. I even planned for them by having two complete sets of wardrobes, each of which were uncomfortable fifty percent of the time, because no one ever goes straight from fat to thin, and I was never thin anyway. Given my sixty-pound variance, I managed to get by with a "skinny" set of slacks, waist sizes 38–40; and a "fat" set, waist sizes 42–44. My XXX shirts batted both ways, and, thankfully, feet don't get fat until the very end. If I was at a point where my clothes were uncomfortably tight, then I just crawled up to the attic and pulled down the giant Tupperware bin labeled "fat clothes." If I was already in my fat clothes, then I just wore XXX surgical scrubs with a 64-inch drawstring that gave me twelve inches on each end to tie a bow, if I cinched it tight enough. I remember a few instances in which I wore tight clothes to work one day and didn't change back into them until months later, when on the undulating down slope of my cyclical obesity, because the thought of squeezing my thunder thighs into dress slacks, like sausage into its casing, was more than I could bear.

Those who are not trying to lose weight

Of all the overweight and obese not trying to lose weight, there are those who hate being fat and those who don't. The ones who hate being fat have given up for the time being; they see no light at the end of the tunnel. Their life circumstances are such that any attempt at weight loss seems hopeless. They have passed under that inscription "Abandon Hope, All Ye Who Enter Here" carved over the doorway to Fat Hell. A goodly portion of these folks are the morbidly obese, previously defined as those one hundred pounds above their ideal body weight, or having a BMI greater than forty. I won't pretend that I can get inside the head of a person in this corpulent condition, but I can get inside my own head without too much difficulty. I can remember brief periods of time when I was morbidly obese and living in the gluttonous third circle of hell—it didn't matter how much I ate, because I was so fat already that it didn't seem like it could get any worse.

I do not think that any morbidly obese person is truly accepting of their obesity, unless they are mentally ill. If anything, there may be unhealthy rationalizations for obesity, one such as—*this is me, this is who I am, I was born this way, I can't help it and, if you love me, you'll have to accept me the way I am.* Nobody likes being obese, and if they say that they do, or don't mind it, they are lying to you and to themselves.

Sadly, the natural progression of a fat person is to become fatter. One of the conveniences of fat is that the more fat there is, the more calories it takes to sustain it. So, when I was three hundred pounds, my daily caloric requirement was 3,000 Calories to remain stable; whereas, at two hundred and fifteen pounds it is a paltry 2,150. Therefore, I can't eat the same amount at 215 as I did at 300 and maintain weight.

Theoretically, there is a point where your body mass might be so great that you could eat as much as you want and not gain any weight, because the metabolic cost of sustaining your corpulence would be so great that there would not be enough hours in the day to eat enough. But then you'd have to get yourself a li'l Rascal, or I should say a big one, because you couldn't walk from here to there, and you'd have to live in a garage on a cement slab because that's the only door you would fit through, and the floor trusses of a conventional home wouldn't support your weight. And then, you'd die.

We all know overweight people who are comfortable with their body habitus and not interested in change, not because they shouldn't be, but because they're not interested in trying. There are even some overweight and obese people who don't think they're overweight or obese, or that it's a problem. They might think that it's a "sexy" fat or a "cute" fat, or that they're not *that* fat. This represents a distorted body image, the opposite of anorexia, and is pathological.

I can identify two specific examples of pathological thinking in regard to my body image. The first one pertained to a dislike of pictures and videos of me because they represented an accurate image of my obesity. I honestly thought that there was some mysterious element of the film that caused me to appear overweight. Of course, the pictures made me look fat *because I was fat.*

The second example of a distorted body image occurred regularly, on Packer Sundays whenever Favre completed a pass to one of his tight ends. The height and weight of the tight end would fill the screen. This was usually along the lines of 6 feet 4 inches and 250–275 lb. "See! See!" I'd say emphatically to Sue. "That could've been me."

Sue didn't share my long-held belief that playing football would have drastically improved our lives, nor did she share a vivid image of me leaping four feet off the ground to pluck Favre's bullet pass out of thin air with buttery-soft hands before bolting across the goal line and Lambeau-leaping into the stands of my adoring fans. Of course, now I realize that I was never even remotely close to the body habitus of an NFL tight end. I recognize my fantasy for what it was—a fantasy, a pathological distortion of body image. With a body fat percentage exceeding thirty percent, this should have been patently obvious to me for the simple reason that the tight end dancing into the end zone, while Favre danced around back at the line of scrimmage, didn't have a round face like me—and he was even on TV, which, at the time, I thought *made people look fat.*

Obesity is a worldwide problem. Civilization is wrestling with an approaching singularity of fat—a battle that it will not win because the singularity requires individual responsibility and action. It cannot be legislated away; it cannot be solved in the courts. If losing weight was easy, then there would be a *minority* of overweight people; alas, it is difficult, and there is a *majority* of overweight people. If you are reading this book, there is a 66 percent chance that you are overweight or obese. Whether you stay where you are or are pulled deeper into the singularity or leave it behind altogether is up to you.

It is only through the collective, individual actions of the overweight and obese that this singularity of fat will be averted. Achieving and maintaining a healthy weight is a matter of balance, and that is what I need to communicate to you. I believe that I can help by sharing with you this not-so-secret *secret* that my patients, acquaintances, and friends are so desperately interested in.

I could share my interpretation of this balance in a cookbook-like list format, but that would be hollow, boring, and meaningless. It is crucial that you understand *why* it is so and *how* it works, and if I can accomplish this with some small measure of pleasure, so much the better. Please let me help you from where you are today to where you would like to be tomorrow. It is a so very interesting journey; with it comes comprehension; with that comes enlightenment; and from enlightenment change follows, as certain as the light of day after the dark of night.

chapter five

The unfairness of fat

I AM SURE THE FAT cell seemed like a good idea to the powers that be in 200,000 BC, but in the 21st century AD, where an energy-dense meal, snack, or drink is only a phone call or few steps away, the fat cell seems much less brilliant. It is as though nearly everything about it is maligned against us in a way that doesn't even seem fair.

The adipocyte, the fat cell—to truly understand it requires a healthy dose of biochemistry. It could be worse. I could have said organic chemistry. Organic chemistry is the bane of pre-med students. It is a John Deere combine equivalent that cuts a wide swath through the annual crops of pre-medical undergraduate students nation-wide. At least biochemistry is somewhat comprehensi-ble. Do you, personally, need to know biochemistry? *Not really.* Do you want to? *Probably not.* This is where I come in. Utilizing my many years of post-graduate training in the health sciences, I am going to interpret and distil, down to a few brief paragraphs, the salient points such that you will gain the power and the knowledge to begin your own journey of enlightenment.

The fat cell is an indulgent cell. It is one of the first places excess energy goes to and generally is the last place energy is released from in attempts to lose weight, if not done in a fairly specific way. The most metabolically active fat is the centrally located visceral fat, which explains why the last place excess body fat is mobilized from is the hips and waist (love handles). The fat cells' primary function is that of energy storage, and our body's physiological goal is to use as little energy as possible at any given time. A prime example of this is during times of fasting and famine—the body senses the decreased caloric intake, and the basal metabolic rate (BMR) is lowered, conserving energy—energy that comes mainly from the adipose tissue stores.

The number of fat cells will never decrease, but they can increase in two instances. The first instance is that of childhood. The number of fat cells will increase throughout childhood, with a final burst of hyperplasia (increase in number) during adolescence. When children and adolescents are overfed, the hyperplasia is accentuated, markedly increasing the number of fat cells and the attendant health risks. Obese children at ages six to nine have a 55 percent chance of becoming obese adults, which is ten times the risk of children with a normal body weight.[15]

The second instance in which fat cells can increase in number is at the extreme end of morbid obesity. As an adult, the number of fat cells is relatively stable in the overfed state, and any increase in body fat mass is due to an increase in the size of the cells. In *mortal* obesity, however, there is again a hyperplasia of fat cells when the finite numbers of cells reach their maximal or finite size. With weight loss there is a decrease in the size of the fat cells, but never a decrease in number, short of surgical removal (liposuction). No amount of weight loss will decrease the total number of fat cells, but they can always increase in number—hardly seems fair, don't you think?

Is it a gland problem? *Rarely.* Is there some biochemical, genetic, or neuroendocrine system that makes me fat? *The biochemical and neuroendocrine systems play a significant part, such as in the role of insulin—the genetic aspect, I feel, is somewhat less significant.* Is it hopeless to even try? Am I meant to be overweight? *Of course not.* Can I do something about it? *Most definitely.*

There is a natural inclination to assign blame for overweight*ness* to something other than self. *Surely, there must be some cause, a medical condition that is responsible for my obesity. Perhaps it's a slow metabolism or some other metabolic defect. It can't be me. I don't eat that much.* During my gradual weight loss, when I plateaued at two-fifty, I became suspicious of a brain tumor because I didn't think I was overeating. I couldn't figure out why I wasn't experiencing headaches, blackouts, or vision changes from the imaginary tumor growing in my brain. It just didn't add up. I wasn't eating an unreasonable amount, and I exercised regularly, in a sporadic sort of way, but still, I couldn't lose any more weight. There had to be something wrong.

If I had a dollar for every normal thyroid panel drawn from the arms of all the overweight and obese in the past twenty years, I don't know if I'd have the time to write this book, because I'd be too busy back rolling off the humongous swim platform of my mega yacht in the tax-free island-nation of Vanuatu. Nonetheless, hypothyroidism is one of the more common secondary causes of obesity, which, when all taken together, are still relatively uncommon. If there is anything on the list below that seems as though it might apply to you, simply take it in to your primary care physician and ask him or her something like—*say, doc, are any of these things etiological (be sure and use this word and he or she will be mightily impressed) in regard to my obesity or overweightness?*

Secondary causes of obesity

- Hypothyroidism: underactive thyroid
- Cushing's syndrome: too much steroid, like from a brain tumor
- Insulinoma: pancreatic tumor
- Hypothalamic obesity: brain problem
- Polycystic ovary syndrome
- Genetic syndromes, of which mental retardation is a common feature: Prader-Willi, Alström, Bardet-Biedl, Cohen, Börjeson-Forssman-Lehmann, and Fröhlich syndromes; if you are reading this, and comprehending it, the likelihood is that you aren't mentally retarded and don't have a genetic syndrome
- Growth hormone deficiency
- Oral contraceptive use
- Pregnancy: this does not mean pregnancy itself, but rather the tendency to gain additional weight over and above that related to fetal weight gain.
- Medication related: phenothiazines (antipsychotics), sodium valproate and carbamazepine (anticonvulsant, bipolar disorder), tricyclic

antidepressants, lithium (bipolar), glucocorti-
coids (steroids), megestrol acetate (appetite-
enhancing drug used in cancer and HIV patients),
thiazolidinediones (treatment of type 2 diabetes,
causes a decrease in leptin level which may lead
to an increased appetite), sulfonylureas (treatment of type 2 diabetes, may cause weight gain
from fluid retention), insulin, adrenergic antagonists (treatment of hypertension, heart disease, enlarged prostate), serotonin antagonists
(cyproheptadine; treatment of allergies and as
appetite stimulant in anorexia nervosa)
- Smoking cessation
- Eating disorders: binge-eating disorder—*guilty,*
  bulimia nervosa—*okay, one time,* night-eating
  disorder—*uh-oh, this is a disorder?*
- Hypogonadism: small testes or ovaries—this is
  an easy one for guys to check, *aah, wait a minute…nope, everything's fine here*
- Pseudohypoparathyroidism: dysfunction of
  small glands by the thyroid

What is the role of genetics in obesity?

The genetic code, sequestered away in billions of strands
of double helix molecules called deoxyribonucleic acid
(DNA), will doom one to a lifetime of obesity in only the
rarest of cases. These rare cases of genetic obesity are
either Mendelian disorders that involve multiple gene
and chromosomal defects, or single gene defects in
which only one segment of the DNA strand is faulty. In
the Mendelian obesity syndromes, obesity is one of several features, including mental retardation, such that if
you are reading this page it would be unlikely that you

are of a Mendelian obese descent. As for the single gene
defects, they are more a problem of mice than of men.
Only one family has been identified with a gene defect
in a hormone, leptin, which is related to appetite regulation; whereas, there are entire lineages of rats and
mice that have exhibited single gene defects resulting in
obesity. Granted, the majority of these arose after some
rather unkind crossbreeding from their human masters;
nonetheless, single gene defects resulting in obesity *in
humans* is exceedingly rare.

Genetics does play a role in the more common forms
of obesity, but it cannot be easily reduced to a biological
defect, such as a missing chromosome or mutation. There
are as many as seventy genes or more that are involved
in body mass, fat distribution, energy uptake, energy
expenditure, and nutrient partitioning. All of these genes
have a variable expression similar to that of height, body
fat pattern, and hair and eye color, which are somewhat
specific to family lines. An easily observable example is
height. A tall parent will have taller children, and two
tall parents will likely have even taller children because
the gene for a greater height is strongly expressed.

The genetic predisposition to overweight and obesity
relating to these inheritable genes can be divided into
two broad categories: a strong genetic predisposition
and a slight genetic susceptibility. The factor common to
both the strong and the slight genetic susceptibility is
that they both require a specific environment (poor eating habits) for the expression of obesity. If, for instance,
you have a child from an obese family line with a genetic
predisposition and poor eating habits who is adopted
into a non-obese family with good eating habits, then

the child is less likely to be obese or overweight than if raised by his or her biological parents.

A study published in the *New England Journal of Medicine* several years ago clearly illustrates a genetic influence on obesity. The researcher overfed twelve pairs of identical twins by a total of 84,000 Calories over the course of one hundred days. The increase in weight was three times more variable between the pairs of unrelated twins as it was between the related siblings—even though all consumed the same amount of excess calories. The twins with identical strands of DNA showed much less variance in weight than those with different strands of DNA. This was a tightly controlled study in which all subjects lived in a dormitory setting and had similar daily energy expenditures, and indeed suggests that there are familial tendencies or a genetic predisposition for weight gain in an overfed state.[16]

So, we know that there can be a genetic predisposition to obesity—what does that mean for me? Do I have a genetic tendency towards obesity? *Possibly.* Genetic screening is available for breast cancer and other conditions. There are already companies that charge a few thousand dollars for sequencing large segments of an individual's genetic code from which certain diseases, like Alzheimer's, might be shown to be of a higher risk. It is likely that in the future genetic screening for obesity will be widely available and as easy as sending in a swab of saliva and a personal check for a few hundred dollars.

The more important question is: what is the result of the test going to change? Is knowing that you have a strong predisposition going to somehow make you less obese? If you are predisposed towards obesity, does that mean that the die is cast and resistance is futile? *Oh no, there's no hope for me now, I may as well continue my descent into Fat Hell and have another ButterBurger with fries on the way down.*

It doesn't matter what the test is.

Predisposition to obesity *does not equal* obesity. You are not meant to be obese.

The environment is the most important aspect of the inheritability of obesity. Genetic factors account for approximately 25 percent of the variation among persons in regards to body fat, but it is the environment that carries the most weight. The definition of "environment" in this instance is thought of as the cultural transmission of lifestyles considered to be "obesogenic."

Having a genetic predisposition to obesity does not mean that you are going to be obese no matter what. It just means that you are more likely to be overweight or obese in an obesogenic environment. It is true that it will be more difficult for those with a genetic predisposition to avoid obesity than it will be for those who have no predisposition. If there is a known predisposition, say a positive test, when available, or a family history of obesity, then one of the chief goals is to realize that potential, accept it, and then institute the proper lifestyle to avoid the slippery slope of obesity.[17,18]

Argument against a genetic role in the current epidemic of obesity

The strongest case against the assignment of blame to genetic factors in regard to the worldwide obesity epidemic is evolution. Evolution does not occur in decades. It occurs in millennia. The epidemiological data referenced in the first section has only been collected over the past fifty years, during which the marked rise in overweight and obesity has been documented. I highly doubt that the human race has evolved towards obesity in that period of time.

Further evidence regarding the evolutionary case is the daguerreotype. Louis-Jacques-Mandé Daguerre invented this earliest form of photography in 1837. A review of online daguerreotypes from 1839–1864 demonstrated one obese and two moderately overweight individuals in the first fifty portraits viewed. Hardly a scientific assessment, I admit; nonetheless, a visually impressive one.

If L.J.M. Daguerre could time-travel to today; take fifty random daguerreotype portraits; time-travel back from whence he came, 150 years ago; and then compare the images, I wonder what he would think. Knowing that he was a contemporary of Charles Darwin, who published *On the Origin of Species* in 1859, perhaps he would have drawn the erroneous conclusion that the human race must have evolved to their present corpulent condition due to the process of natural selection. He may have concluded that an ice age must be fast approaching and that the human race evolved to the extra fat for warmth. L.J.M. Daguerre would have been wrong. Even Darwin's finches required a few generations to change the color of their feathers. The round faces in the images from the future were primarily of an environmental cause, not a genetic one.

Leptin

I will discuss only one of the fat genes, *obese*, notated as "*ob*." It is a gene that is active in adipose tissue, allowing for the synthesis of leptin, which is a hormone responsible for satiety. *Leptin* is derived from the Greek word *leptos*, which means thin. It has many actions throughout the body, but one of its main effects is in the brain, where it acts upon a part of the brain called the hypothalamus to suppress the appetite. It tells your brain that you should stop eating when your caloric intake is maintaining the ideal fat stores. The serum concentration of leptin is proportionate to the amount of adipose tissue—the more fat there is, the higher the leptin levels are in the bloodstream.

The problem in obesity is not a lack of leptin but, rather, a resistance to it. A tolerance develops, just like any other drug, such as alcohol or morphine—if you are exposed to it often enough and in increasing amounts, it takes more and more of it to have an effect. This is directly analogous to the elevated insulin levels in type 2 diabetes and insulin resistance. In obese individuals there are elevated levels of leptin, and therefore a relative leptin resistance of the tissues, including the hypothalamus. As a result, the feedback mechanism, in the hypothalamus, becomes increasingly more resistant to leptin and it takes more and more leptin to tell the brain to stop eating, with the end result being chronic overeating. This is well documented by studies demonstrating that elevated leptin levels correlate with central obesity, glucose intolerance, hypertriglyceridemia and hypertension.

It has also been demonstrated that weight loss lowers leptin levels, causing a decrease in tissue resistance; and weight gain increases the blood levels, causing an increase in tissue resistance. We can surmise, therefore, that leptin resistance, as insulin resistance, is reversible with weight loss and with the establishment of proper, long-term dietary patterns and lifestyle modifications that are addressed in the upcoming second and third pillars.[19,20,21]

Set point theory

The set point theory holds that obesity results from a metabolic defect, which allows for a variation of the basal metabolic rate to maintain weight at a "set point." It suggests that when an obese person loses weight, their metabolic rate slows down and energy is conserved until the weight is regained (*this is not the same as the slowing of the metabolic rate as part of the fasting response mentioned earlier*). This thought is prevalent in the healthcare field, as well as in the general public, as it is consistent with the high recidivism rate of obesity—only a minority of dieters keep their weight off for an extended period of time.

The set point theory as stated is a fallacy. Your metabolic rate does not change with weight loss in order to maintain a set point (weight). This has been validated by sophisticated studies in which different groups of overweight people were compared—those who regained weight after losing it, and those who were able to maintain weight loss. The only significant difference between those who maintained weight loss and those who didn't was the level of daily energy expenditure. That is to say, those who were more sedentary did not tend to maintain weight loss—*there was not a slowing of the basal metabolic rate in those who regained weight.*[22,23]

If there is a set point, it is a psychological set point or an environmental set point, and this needs to be "reset" with a healthy dose of education, which we are about, and behavioral modification, which we will accomplish.

Is there a viral cause of obesity?

If you recall from the earlier part of this chapter, I made
the point that fat cells can increase in number in only two
situations: in childhood, and at the extreme end of obesity when the fat cells can't get any bigger. Unfortunately,
it seems that there is likely a third way. In January of
2009 there was a brief flurry of coverage of a "fat virus"
in the lay media. Every news outlet ran with the story
until it was bumped back out of awareness by something
else. I'm not sure why it was in the news that particular day because the studies that addressed the question
of a virus as a potential etiological agent for obesity
were published a number of years ago—a couple of the
definitive human studies being done in 2005.

There have been several viruses that have been
shown to cause obesity in animals, but, to date, in
humans there seems to be only one—the human adenovirus. There are more than fifty different types of the
adenovirus, which is implicated in up to ten percent of
upper respiratory tract infections in children and adults.
That's right. The fat virus is a cousin of the common cold
virus, if not the cold virus itself. *Ah-CHEW! Oh, excuse me;
I must have caught a lifetime of obesity.*

The specific adenovirus implicated is Ad-36 and the
evidence for its link to obesity can be found in three key
studies. The first human study, from 2005, tested 502
individuals for Ad-36 and found that 30 percent of obese
individuals tested positive, while in a matching population, only 11 percent of lean individuals tested positive.
The separation in weight between the two groups was an
average of 9 units of BMI.[24] For instance, assuming that I
am seronegative (test negative) for Ad-36, at a height and

weight of 75 inches and 220 lb. my BMI is 27. That means that in a parallel universe where I am seropositive (test positive) for Ad-36, my BMI is 36 with a weight of around 290. This represents a difference of 70 pounds, which is surprisingly close to my obesogenic past, which causes me to wonder if I am seropositive already? *Hmmm.*

The second key human study was conducted in 89 twin pairs in which both twins were tested for Ad-36. In the twin pairs where one twin tested positive and the other negative, there was a small but significant difference in weight. The seropositive twins were significantly fatter than their seronegative siblings. Although the difference was significant, it was small, with only about 1.5 units of BMI separation, and a measured 2 percent increase in body fat of the seropositive twin.[24] This association is much less impressive than the first referenced study, with the difference in weight being only 10–15 pounds (1.5 units of BMI), as opposed to the 70-pound difference of those in the first study who did not share the same genetic code.

The third key human study involved the direct inoculation of human stem cells with Ad-36. In this case, the "infected" stem cells showed both an increased tendency to differentiate into fat cells and an increased tendency to increase fat storage as compared to "non-infected" stem cells.[25] The increased tendencies were shown to be enhanced with both an increasing viral load, and the passage of time.

It is clear that there is an association of Ad-36 and obesity; however, is it a causal relationship? *Does the fat virus actually cause obesity?* I'm afraid so. In addition to the above-referenced human study suggesting causation, there were also multiple animal studies preceding it which demonstrated a specific gene within the virus that induced both *an increase* in fat accumulation within the cells *and an increase* in the number of fat cells.[26]

The larger question is, now what? What if I am seropositive for Ad-36? Should I be tested? Does this mean that I might already be doomed to a lifetime of obesity?

I would suggest that as long as there is no vaccine or specific treatment, then it doesn't really matter. What would it change if you knew? Despite the studies suggesting a causative relationship, given the difference in the above first two studies looking at the association, my sense is that there may be more of an association than there is a cause. I think that the significance of the fat virus is that those who are positive *may* have a more difficult time at maintaining weight loss; but, it is certainly nothing that a proper outlook and lifestyle changes can't overcome. Like a genetic predisposition, seropositivity for Ad-36 is currently out of our control, other than living in a sterile bubble, and therefore requires acceptance and adaptation. Both genetic predisposition and Ad-36 seropositivity do not automatically a fat person make. They only imply susceptibility. They can be overcome. I will tell you how.

Why is fat good, other than chocolate, steak, and ice cream?

Energy, young man, energy!

The main components of our diet are carbohydrates, fat, and protein. All of these ingested nutrients that are not utilized for activities or bodily functions are converted into triglycerides in the adipocyte (fat cell). In the fasting state the triglycerides are hydrolyzed (react with water) into glycerol and fatty acids. Fatty acids are a major source of fuel and when metabolized they yield more than twice the energy of carbohydrates or protein per unit weight—nine Calories per gram, as opposed to four Calories per gram.

The amount of triglyceride residing in the fat cells of the normal average adult human is about 25 lb and sufficient to maintain life for forty days and forty nights; like, maybe in a desert? Hmmm...what a coincidence, *or is it?*

I found this little nugget of information in my *bible* of biochemistry, *Textbook of Biochemistry with Clinical Correlations,* by Thomas M. Devlin, copyright 1982. I hadn't cracked that particular volume in the past twenty years. It only said forty days. I added the forty nights and the desert part, recognizing the biblical implications, because, if you have forty days, logically, there are forty following nights, unless you don't count the last one, in which case there are only thirty-nine. I counted it for the impact. Wow!

Now that we have a better understanding of over-weight*ness,* let us move on to the good stuff. The following three sections form a trinity, as I've come to think about it these past few years. I have organized them in order of importance. The first pillar of the triad, *emotional health*, involves some scientific building blocks that have applications in the latter two pillars, *diet and energy* and *energy expenditure.*

The primary goal of this book is to bring about a change in you as significant as what I have experienced on a personal level. A component of this change will be weight loss; however, in order for that to occur long term, there must follow other changes as well. I feel that this can only occur through the transmission of knowledge. I can't just tell you what to do—that wouldn't last. It never does. You need to know *why,* and *how* it is so. Therein lies your empowerment—your *enlightenment.*

EMOTIONAL HEALTH

Those who are not shocked when they first come across quantum mechanics cannot possibly have understood it.

Niels Bohr

I cannot believe that God would choose to play dice with the universe.

Albert Einstein

Einstein, don't tell God what to do.

Neils Bohr

The theory of quantum electrodynamics describes Nature as absurd from the point of view of common sense...So I hope you can accept Nature as She is—absurd.

Richard Feynman

You mean there's a parallel universe where Wylie E. Coyote *catches* the Road Runner?

Shaun Melarvie

chapter six

A revelation

THE REVELATION OF A cohesive strategy in which to achieve a lifelong, stable, and appropriate BMI occurred to me several months ago in the Catholic church of Corpus Christi. It happened during Father Tony's homily. I don't know for what reason, but I was looking at the mural, to the right of the nave, of the Virgin Mary, who was cradling a prostrate Jesus, freshly deceased. A dove, encased in rays of light, hovered over Mary's right shoulder. Behind me, a baby cried. At that moment, the revelation seeped into my consciousness, as the rising sun illuminates the eastern sky. I cannot say with any certainty that my newfound awareness was related in any way to Father's words, but I can say that my mind was open, as it seems to be during much of the Mass.

Sue was sitting on my left, nestled in my outstretched arm resting on the back of the pew, which was our customary sitting position. We were holding hands, her right in my left. She wore a tanzanite ring on the third finger, above her wedding band. I bought it for her in St. Thomas for our 25th wedding anniversary that was still ten years away, but it made it easier to justify the not inconsiderable expenditure of twenty-eight hundred dollars at the time. I tilted my head towards her ear and breathed softly, "Trinity."

She looked at me thinking, I'm sure, *what's he talking about*, and so I added, "An idea, remind me after church." As though I'd forget—it occupied my thoughts all through the Eucharist prayer, which is the part of Mass where I generally do my deepest thinking. The Eucharist prayer is in the mid-portion of Mass, preceded by the offertory, which is notable for a few parishioners, preferably a family, who take the bread and wine up to Father Tony, standing in the center of the nave along with Deacon Paul and the servers. Other than the consecration of the Host, the Eucharist prayer is remarkable for the time spent on our knees, which I believe is specific to the Catholic fraction of Christians.

After the congregation drops collectively to bended knees, Father performs some preliminaries and then embarks on either a mercifully short Eucharist prayer where he pretty much cuts to the...*this is my body...this is my blood*...part; or a less merciful medium or long version where numerous saints' and popes' names are brought up, with other elaborations, that seems to drag on eternally such that when I stand up I expect to see blood soaking through my slacks due to bilateral pressure ulcerations from my tibial tuberosities—those lumps on the bone below the kneecaps. It has been my experience that the length of the prayer is inversely proportional to the length of the homily, unless it's Packer Sunday, and then both are short.

Years ago, during the consecration portion of the Eucharist prayer, when the bread and wine are changed to the body and blood of Christ, tiny little bells would ring twice: once, just before "this is my body," and a second time just before "this is my blood." So, although it was possible for the inattentive to miss the first half of the consecration, rarely did they miss the second half. For several years now, there has been no prepubescent altar boy ringing the cloverleaf-like arrangement of little silver bells heralding the consecration, but I somehow still hear their crisp tinkle in my head. No matter how deep in thought I am, related or unrelated to God, I never missed that part; except for that one particular Sunday when I first thought of the Trinity in an unchristian way.

The Trinity—the Father, the Son and the Holy Ghost— represents the three pillars of the Christian faith. Over the past several months as I've thought of writing my epistle, which is how I initially thought of it, I have struggled with the structure, with what I wanted to say and how to say it. On a Sunday, in the middle of Father Tony's sermon, the third and most important pillar of the Diet Theory of Everything was delivered into my consciousness—emotional health.

My wife and I have been on many diets—all the major ones—Sue even more so than I, because there are some things that even I wouldn't eat for more than two days in a row. We tried variations of the *lose ten pounds in one week* diet, such as the cabbage soup diet, the all the fruit and vegetables you can eat diet, and many others long since forgotten.

Guess what?

They worked. We would lose ten or more pounds in one week. We felt good about ourselves. We would celebrate by slipping into smaller-sized Calvin Kleins that would mysteriously shrink over the course of the following week, as surely as if a witch doctor in a grass skirt and nose ring and dancing around a fire deep in the Congo had cast an evil spell.

The inconvenient truth of these various diets is that they didn't work for long and we eventually gained our weight back, be it days, weeks, or months later. In some cases we gained back more weight than we lost. Long-term weight loss remained an elusive goal always in sight but unattainable, like a far-off, hazy mountain that never gets closer, forever receding into the distance with any attempt to approach it.

But that was then; this is now—now being the past four years that Sue and I have had a stable weight with a healthy BMI. We have changed our lives by implementing lifestyle changes that allow for a proper balance between the three pillars of the Diet Theory of Everything: emotional health, diet and energy, and energy expenditure. If you could pick only one of the triad to address, I would pick the first one, emotional health, because I feel that would carry you the farthest along the path you must travel.

Anyone can lose weight in the short term by diet alone or by exercise alone or a combination thereof. We have all done this at some point in the past, but it was and is doomed to failure without the proper balance between the three components of the trinity. This balanced approach is the means by which you can achieve a wholesome and healthy lifestyle that a normal BMI is only part of.

Defining emotional health

In my attempt at addressing such a broad topic of emotional health, please understand that it is only that—an attempt. An entire encyclopedia, from A to Z, would not be sufficient to adequately address the topic in its entirety. All that I can hope to do is to cause you to think and to wonder of a possibility—the possibility and probability of a better life. What I am going to share represents my impressions and feelings. I would not be so presumptuous as to suggest that I have all the answers; but I do feel that I have some of the answers—enough such that I was able to effect a significant, long-lasting, positive change in my life. What I am going to share with you is the way I see our place in our reality. This is what has made a difference to me. Perhaps it will make a difference to you as well.

People are overweight or obese for many reasons. It might be the bartender in a Mexican restaurant who munches all day long on hazelnuts he floats on top of blended margaritas, and who tosses back the leftovers in the bottom of the blender after making Pink Squirrels and Golden Cadillacs—*okay, this was me, working my 4*th *and 5*th *undergraduate years for $3.75/hr.* It could be the all you can eat, of whatever you want, three times a day meal plan that brings your dorm-bound college student home for Christmas break twenty pounds heavier—*me again, first three years of undergrad.* It could be that the reason is as simple as the combination of readily available, energy-dense foods and poor judgment, but I would intimate that it may be more complex than that.

One area of difficulty to overcome is that our current-day diet is not our natural diet—it will take a few million years for that to happen. Our bodies have not yet evolved to the variety and easy availability of energy-dense food. The physiology of modern man is not at all modern. Our physiology is that of the Neanderthal who chased his next meal a couple of miles over rough terrain before dragging it back to the family cave to eat it raw, along with a bushel of plant fiber that probably had a higher caloric cost of consumption than that contained within its cellular structure. Obviously, we are not going to walk into the wilderness without a camp stove, armed with only a knife, but we would benefit from an understanding of our metabolism and how our body processes the different types of food that we eat.

The convenient truth is that the great majority of us have the power to live and eat in such a fashion as to allow a *healthy* BMI. Now I understand the natural tendency of taking the path of least resistance, which I am well acquainted with. I understand the "id" of—if it feels good, do it—if it tastes good, eat it. But, as humans, endowed as we are with freedom of choice, *why do so many of us choose to be overweight?*

The answer to the question of why so many of us choose to be overweight may be as simple as a poor understanding of caloric need and the energy density of food, which is easy enough to address; or the answer may be as complex as the first triad of our trinity, emotional health, which may not be as prone to disentanglement.

Of course there are different answers for different people, but for some people food is a comfort. It fills a hole, an emptiness, rather than filling a daily caloric need. This is not obvious to those filling that hole. It was not obvious to me. Sure, there were the holidays and other periodic celebrations *of whatever,* in which I knew that I overate, but in general I felt that my intake was not unreasonable. I didn't identify that I was eating from undue anxiety, repressed anger, post-traumatic stress or some other aspect of ill health. All I could really say is that if I wasn't munching, nibbling, sucking, or chewing on something, I wasn't quite comfortable. I was not able to recognize the significance of a lack of emotional health until I was actually in possession of it.

In choosing to not be overweight, it is essential to be emotionally healthy. *What does that mean? How do I even know if I am emotionally unhealthy?* These are tough questions that are subject to a very subjective interpretation. It all depends on who you ask. Each of us needs to take the responsibility to find out the answers on our own, perhaps at times assisted by constructive and compassionate guidance of whichever source.

It is important that we share an acceptable, common understanding of what emotional health, or the lack thereof, might be. *Are you happy? Do you find yourself smiling for no specific reason? Do you feel good about yourself?* In keeping it simple, I suppose we could define "emotional health" as being happy more than half the time. In addition to identifying the presence of emotional health, it might be helpful to identify its absence, which might be reflected by negative emotional states, such as anger or sadness, and unhealthy dysfunctional behaviors.

I think that we can all identify periods in our lives of all of these things; happiness, sadness, and unhealthy choices. But, what has been the emotional course of your life over time? Whether you are chronically happy or chronically sad most likely has more to do with history than with more recent events. Acute happiness or sadness is typically a reaction to a temporally related event, such as the Packers winning the NFC championship game, or losing the Super Bowl. Most people have been the way they are for quite some time, a product of decades of history. As personality traits are established very early in life, difficulty in these years may lead to manifestations of psychopathology in later years. Adults who have emotional issues may be dealing with a problem that has a source within their family of origin rather than within a current relationship.

The world is full of dysfunctional people and dysfunctional families. I suspect that dysfunction is much like our epidemic of overweight and obesity in that there are more who are dysfunctional than are not, such that it almost seems normal to be dysfunctional. Having only recently become slightly less dysfunctional than I used to be, I wonder if an ideal family, or a functional family, really exists in our society today. Perhaps a more realistic goal would be to become only less dysfunctional, which may be the best our human nature can accomplish.

What is dysfunctional? That sounds bad. I feel that to be emotionally healthy is our default human condition. We are meant to be happy, like a child. If we are not, then something has happened. Something has happened to change us from a happy person to a sad one; therefore, dysfunction could be defined as patterns of behavior that keep us from our chronic state of being open to the possibility of happiness. Obvious examples of dysfunctional behavior would be those associated with the common addictions of drugs, alcohol, gambling, pornography, shopping, and food. The secondary effects of these dysfunctional patterns of behavior could include criminal activity, spousal abuse, loss of job, ill health, obesity, financial hardship, and other negative consequences.

The difficulty one encounters in any attempt to harness these dysfunctional patterns is that they feel good at the time. It is the consequences that may be painful. It's like we're the rat pulling a lever in a B. F. Skinner laboratory experiment; only, instead of a treat, we get the potential for pain. Our transient reward is pulling the lever—it feels good at the time, or at least we think it does.

Are we sad because we're dysfunctional or are we dysfunctional because we're sad? Where is the primacy?

Dysfunctional behavior results in negative feelings that reinforce further dysfunctional behavior. Where that dysfunction comes from is the more crucial question; this is where an individual's history becomes pertinent. Dysfunction begets dysfunction. It is cyclical and passed on from parent to child, like blond hair and blue eyes, except that it is a cultural transmission rather than a genetic one. Unlike the genetic transmission of a physical trait that is beyond one's control, the transmission of dysfunction is vulnerable to one's knowledgeable intervention. It is within your control to interrupt it or stop it.

Although it is possible that dysfunction can be traced back to one traumatic episode of emotional abuse, more likely, it is related to a lifetime of experiences of emotional harm. There is physical abuse and there is emotional abuse; however, I am focusing on the emotional, because that is what is ultimately at the root of all dysfunction. In most cases one will recover from the physical abuse—wounds heal—but it is the emotional injury from that physical assault that has a lasting impact. Emotional injury can be acute and blatant or chronic and insidious or any combination thereof. The collective result is the same—emotional damage, always—physical damage, sometimes. Regardless of the pattern of injury, the excreta can be distilled down to two general origins of dysfunctional behavior: low self-worth—*you don't love yourself enough*, and narcissism—*you love yourself too much.*

It is your responsibility to break the cycle—for yourself, for your children, and for your children's children. Breaking the cycle of dysfunctional behavior does not only involve that from parent to child, but also from adult child to parent, if a dysfunctional unhealthy relationship exists. As an adult, you no longer require a parent's support for the basic necessities of life; therefore, if a parent is a cause of emotional pain, then it is your choice to remove that cause. You might choose to sever the relationship altogether, or you might choose to redefine that relationship with an appropriate set of boundaries.

You cannot expect to break another's pattern of dysfunctional behavior. That is their burden, just as your dysfunctional behavior is your burden. There are those who can provide guidance, love and support, but ultimately, the duty of interrupting your dysfunctional behavior must fall on your shoulders alone. *Can you undo all the injustices done to you?* Of course not. *Do they even matter now?* Only if you let them.

How can I break the cycle of dysfunctional behavior?

Breaking the cycle of dysfunctional behavior is difficult. It means that you must diverge from the path of least resistance. It is human nature to take the path of least resistance because, well, there's less resistance.

It's easier. This applies to both our physical lives and our emotional lives.

What takes more effort, going for a two-mile walk after dinner, or sinking into a welcoming sofa to watch TV with a bag of microwaved popcorn that only takes a couple of minutes to make? What takes more effort, writing down or making a physical record of your calories for the day, or making a mental note that you're sure to forget by the end of the day?

What takes more effort, discussing something hurtful that a friend or significant other said to you, or letting it slide? What takes more effort, nursing an anger or resentment for sometimes a very long time, or taking the direct action of forgiving and letting it go? *Hmmm, that's a tough one.* I think that it would take much more effort to feed and water a resentment like a distasteful potted plant for years and years than it would take to just let it go.

We are at a place in our lives from which we wish to move. It is time to take the path less traveled. It is time to break the cycle. I would appreciate your tolerance of the occasional religious overtones throughout the book as they are simply reflections of me. You will find that my ideas are equally viable with a more secular interpretation, if that is what you would be more comfortable with. With that in mind, a good start in cycle-breaking in regard to dysfunctional behavior would be the avoidance of sin.

Man is by nature a sinful creature. Catholicism tells us that we are born into sin—barred forever from the heavenly gates without the sanctification of the sacrament of Baptism. We sin unto others and they unto us.

None are without sin. We have all cast stones. Perhaps "sin" is not the most useful word, as it implies religiosity, and is possibly not applicable to an agnostic; therefore, let me use the word "flagitiousness." I don't recall ever running across that word in the Bible so it might more aptly apply to both the believer and nonbeliever alike.

I think that we all understand the concept of flagitiousness and if not, recognizing what some flagitiousnesses are might be instructive. So let us identify the seven deadly flagitiousnesses, thought to have been set forth by the fourth-century monk Evagrius Ponticus: lust, gluttony, greed, sloth, wrath, envy, and pride. *Uh-oh— Houston, we have a problem.* I've committed all of these sins at least once a week on any given Packer Sunday considering my exposure to scantily clad cheerleaders, bowls of Doritos, enticing commercials stimulating want and desire, anger with losses, pride with wins, and not bothering to put on my pretty after getting out of bed in the morning.

I think that it is safe to say that we can all relate to the seven deadly sins in one way or another. I also think that it is safe to say that from a secular sense they are as undesirable as they are from a religious sense, and by a secular sense, I mean the Judeo-Christian values that our society is based upon. As for myself, I cannot help but think of them in the religious sense because that is how I was brought up.

I remember that time of the sacrament of Reconciliation and Holy Communion, which were sandwiched somewhere between Easter and the summer break that followed second grade. The sacrament of Reconciliation happened so quickly that I scarce remember it; apparently a necessity slipped in just before Holy Communion so that my seven-year-old soul would be ready to receive the body and blood of Christ. It is only because of their close proximity that I must recount them simultaneously.

I remember that first taste of the just-consecrated Host on a Sunday morning in front of the congregation—dry, and then sticky—a taste unlike any other, but pleasing; maybe like a cross between white Wonder bread and an unsalted cracker. I remember that I liked it, and that I wished it were possible for me to have more, so that I could eat them one after another, like a bag of potato chips. Over the following years, I swallowed hundreds of Hosts, given my parochial school exposure to daily Mass, and I often wondered if the priests didn't snack on bags of unconsecrated wafers, because I figured that's what I would have done if I were a priest.

The neurons in my brain containing the taste of unleavened bread must be the very same ones or at least are immediately adjacent to the ones containing trepidation for the confessional, because a recollection of one invariably triggers a recollection of the other. Every subsequent visit to the confessional, after that first one, even as an adult, brings back those very first memories of the awareness of sin, and the weight of sin—the sense of having done something bad that is somehow reflected in the state of a soul, which as a child meant something akin to black spots on an otherwise white as freshly fallen snow soul. Those words, whispered in the dark, are like a time machine to 1968, with the only difference being the number and size of the black spots.

Bless me, Father, for I have sinned. It has been a lifetime since my last confession, as this is my first one. Okay, I admit I didn't say that my first time, although it would have sounded pretty precocious. Maybe Einstein would have said something like it if he had been Catholic.

Forgive me for hitting my sister…for not listening to my mom and dad…and for thinking mean things about my friend, Tony.

I forget exactly what Father said, other than something about a couple of Our Fathers, an act of contrition, and some Hail Marys; but I do remember the soft hiss of the wooden shade closing off the window in my confessional. I felt the release at that very instant, along with a small empathetic shiver for the poor little bastard on the other side. That sound of polished wood sliding on crushed velvet was the sound of release—a release from the weight of sin, and a release from the dark confines of the confessional.

As a Catholic, my trips to the confessional, as well as my church attendance, are not the ideal, but still, my post-confessional feeling is not that far removed from that of 1968, which I find a little curious because what difference does it make if I ask God directly for forgiveness, or an intermediary, even if a priest, and even if, as a Catholic, I'm supposed to believe that it does make a difference? I guess—that's just me being Catholic—and whether you choose to think of flagitiousness in the religious sense as I do, or in the secular sense, as a construct of Greco-Roman morality, it doesn't much matter as long as the end result is similar, that being the avoidance of sin.

Do not be flagitious. This would be a good starting point in breaking the cycle of dysfunctional behavior. Consider the golden rule—do unto others as you would have them do unto you. Consider the last five of the Ten Commandments carved into the second of the stony tablets that Moses carried down from Mount Sinai in 1300 BC. They are secular and do not mention God.

Five—Honor thy father and mother.
Six—Thou shall not kill.
Seven—Thou shall not commit adultery.
Eight—Thou shall not steal.
Nine—Thou shall not bear false witness against thy neighbor.
Ten—Thou shall not covet anything that is thy neighbor's.

It is in this spirit of "to do good things," implied by these commandments and the golden rule, that the morality of Western civilization is founded upon. Therefore, start here. This is your task—to do good things. You don't even have to believe in God, or in going to confession, although you are free to do so. It is a matter of choice, as is everything else.

On being sad

The world is filled with tragedy. It has lived in all of us, if we've lived long enough. It is inescapable, and *everyone* has some manner of a cross to bear; my father abandoned me, my mother died of cancer when I was only seven, my mother's boyfriend raped me, I lost my leg in the war, I was beaten as a child, my sister committed suicide, my home was repossessed, I killed my best friend while driving drunk, my child died from leukemia. And so it goes, from the beginning of human existence as it will until the end of it.

It is obvious that all of these things are tragic and to list them one after another is almost desensitizing and subtracts from the intense pain and grief that an individual or family experiences with any one of these unfortunate examples. My only point is that the commonality of tragedy is that it is spoken of in the past tense. This means that it is not happening or about to happen, but, rather, it has already happened. In living our lives one day at a time, as we do, what purpose is there in allowing sadness from the past to color each new day of the rest of our earthly existence in shades of grey? You can think bad thoughts and relive bad memories over and over, all day long, for a lifetime; but being trapped in the past soils the present and defeats the future.

In Elisabeth Kübler-Ross's book *On Death and Dying*, she identifies five stages of grief: denial, anger, bargaining, depression, and acceptance. Whenever something tragic happens to us, we experience the feelings associated with these stages, perhaps in no particular order, other than acceptance hopefully coming at the end. The important thing, I think, is to recognize these difficult, initial stages as temporary and to continue moving forward, rather than becoming stuck in a pattern of anger, denial or depression. I understand that this is an incredibly sensitive and complex subject, far outside of the scope of this book, but, ultimately, whether it be days, weeks, or months, or however long it takes to work through these emotional stages, the healthy stage to be in after a period of misfortune is that of *acceptance*.

I have implied that there is emotional harm at the root of all dysfunctional behavior—that all dysfunctional people have been victims. This implication suggests that we all are born with an innate goodness that somehow becomes corrupted by a harmful environment. But…

What if you can't remember any abuse? What if there is no smoking gun? First of all, just because you don't remember significant emotional injury doesn't mean that it didn't happen. Secondly, it doesn't really matter— let's just say that you are *not* a victim. As long as you recognize destructive behavior and begin the process of healing yourself, the past becomes relatively irrelevant in a hurry.

I wish that I could simply give a simple command, such as "be happy from this day forward," and it would be so. I am afraid that nothing is that easy, unless it has to do with gravity and falling to earth. Unfortunately, I am not a genie, or a deity, and my simple command is not likely to create happiness. You have to learn how to give happiness and health to yourself, and that could involve some fairly heavy lifting.

A major step towards that goal is the act of forgiveness. Forgiveness goes both ways. If you have been a victim, you must let go of residual anger and bitterness and forgive those who have caused you harm. The emotional baggage is of no use to you.

If you have been a perpetrator of flagitiousness, you must accept responsibility for your actions, face the consequences, and seek forgiveness from those you have harmed. You may or may not be forgiven in the human realm, but, at the end of the day, *you need to forgive yourself.*

Some will not be able to pull themselves from the hole of their past and will need professional help, or at least the compassionate support of close friends or a significant other. I wish that there were something I could write, a magic word or a powerful phrase, that would unlock a door in a troubled mind and make it all better. Although I have no magic word, I can say that I have traveled a definite path to health and happiness.

This is where I am trying to lead you. If you look—around you are happy and successful people, the kind that are smiling and effervescent such that you have to smile in return, the kind who brighten a room by their very presence. These people have not been magically free of suffering. They too have suffered, as has everyone in our human condition. The key difference is that they have made the conscious decision to stop—*suffering*.

Just as there is effort in maintaining a virtuous life, in abiding by the golden rule, and the secular commandments, there is also effort in maintaining a joyous life. Joy will not drop from the sky in a perpetual drizzle. Joy is only ephemeral. You must open your life to the possibility of it. There will continue to be tragedy. That is the nature of the world in which we live. It is the sadness in our lives that accents the happiness. It is a necessary contrast. If the minimum definition of happiness is the absence of sadness, how could we possibly experience one without the other?

It may be that you are already happy and emotionally healthy. That would be very nice. If not, I hope that I may have triggered some contemplation of the state of your own emotional health. What I am suggesting is that if you can identify a problem, and wrap your mind about it, then you are well on your way to solving it. It is time to empower yourself, through an awareness of self, to change yourself for the better as you travel your own pathway to enlightenment.

Perhaps your path will involve professional psychotherapy. Perhaps your path will be a personal journey of self-discovery, facilitated by the process of keeping a daily journal. I know a man who wrote letters to his deceased mother because it was important for him to think his thoughts out loud—he needed to get them out of his head and onto the paper in front of him; it was only then that he could deal with them.

You might declare this day a new day and cast off your burdensome cloak of tragedy. *Why?* Because you can. It is in your power. You can make the conscious decision to do good things, to treat others as you would like yourself to be treated. You can make the conscious decision to stop suffering. Replace a frown with a smile. Replace a negative thought with a positive one. At least once a year, perhaps on the anniversary of your new day, live that one day as if it were your last. *What would you do differently? Who would you call and talk to?*

chapter seven

Positive energy

AS I'VE SAID, EMOTIONAL health is the important part. It is actually the hardest part, but it matters most. Weight loss is often only the by-product of being emotionally healthy. Now, just because you can't identify dysfunctional behavior doesn't mean that it isn't there, but for the sake of argument let us say that it isn't. Let us assume that you are already emotionally healthy and happy. If that is the case, feel free to skip ahead to the second pillar. However, *is there such a thing as being too emotionally healthy? Can you be too happy?* We have a saying in surgery that "the enemy of good is better." This does not apply to emotional health. No matter how emotionally healthy you are, or aren't, you can *always* be better.

Being happy is nothing more than *being in a state of relativity.* Whichever happiness frame of reference we are in at any one time, you need to understand that it is only that—a relative frame of reference, from which we will move into another. Now, our task is to understand how we can move up the relativity scale of being happy, and how we can recover from those inevitable periods of sadness that we all experience throughout our lives. Our task is to understand how to do this by a logical application of truth and the natural laws of our universe. Like happiness, being emotionally healthy is only a relative state, with a lesser state and a greater state on either side of it.

Hopefully, I've goaded you into completing the second part of the first pillar of our triad, because this is the part of my path to enlightenment that I enjoyed the most. From the chapter title "Positive Energy," you may infer that I am going to spend all of our time on positive thinking, positive mental imagery, and looking into a mirror and saying, "How are you doing today, self? Gee, you look terrific." That is not the case.

I believe in the power of an amalgam of what I loosely refer to as positive energy. Before you can truly understand the power of positive energy, it is first necessary to understand the universe. Okay, maybe not really, really understand it, but at least to have an inkling of it, how it fits together and the significance of positive energy in whichever form, because, at the end of the day, life is mostly about probability, and the goal is to be happy more often than sad. Positive energy is a powerful tool to realizing that goal.

There are people exponentially smarter than me who could explain the universe with lines of complex mathematical equations, string theory, and daring propositions of the theory of everything, but you'd have to be smart, like them, to comprehend their genius. Not being one of these people, I've been reduced to merely reading.

I have always been a voracious reader. I can spend an infinite amount of time in any bookstore, or a book section of any store. I have read every genre of fiction, including the adult western, which I discovered one memorable afternoon in the Owl Bookstore in Bismarck, North Dakota. *I suspect this may have been my first violation of the first deadly sin.* I was fifteen at the time and the author was Jake Logan. His protagonist, Jake Slocum, was a brawny, virile cowboy who I could relate to because I felt fairly virile myself, in a frustrated sort of way, and if not as brawny as Jake Slocum I was at least brawnier than most of my peers.

I didn't notice the fairly obvious red emblem on the cover that identified the novel as an adult western, but before I turned the first steamy page, I knew that this was a far cry from Zane Grey or Louis L'Amour—this was special, and unlike any western I had ever read before. Over the course of my summer break, I read all of the Jake Slocum westerns that I could find at the Owl, violating the first deadly sin over and over again until I imagined my once Casper-white soul as being a mottled sable from a veritable blizzard of sticky, black snowballs of sin. Twenty years later I came across a worn, dog-eared copy of a Jake Slocum novel at a rummage sale. I picked it up and ran my finger across the tattered, glossy cover—*A Noose for Slocum.* Only then did I realize the obvious play on his name.

Somewhere along the course of my journey to an appropriate BMI my reading tastes abruptly matured. If I had to point to a specific moment in which this change occurred, I would have to say that it was during another, less memorable afternoon in Barnes & Noble when I threw a copy of *The Elegant Universe*, by Brian Green, on a stack of bargain-priced books that I took up to the counter. This was the first nonfiction book, outside of my education, that I had ever purchased, apart from *Life and Death in a Coral Sea*, by Jacques Cousteau. Since that moment, three years ago, I have been reading nonstop, the only fiction being two novels, required by my book club—everything else has been nonfiction.

Introduction to quantum physics— from Homer to Hemingway: why happiness = mc²

I feel the need to preface the next few chapters with a warning of sorts. I don't know why I am so interested— perhaps obsessed *would be a better word—in a subject about which I know so little. My only hope is that I will be able to convey some sense of the mystery and beauty of our universe; and if not, then at least I tried.*

Please, don't worry about trying to understand or grasp everything that you read. Please don't let your eyes glaze over, causing you to set aside the book. Please, breathe deep, get a cup of coffee, and then read on. Please forgive me that which I've explained poorly and enjoy that which I've explained more adequately; and if not even that, then enjoy the funny part in the middle. Good luck.

A few areas of concentration in my reading have been physics and classical Greece. I don't know why I wasn't as fascinated about these things in high school and college as I am now. I suppose it was a chore back then, a ticket to get punched on my card of life that would allow a respectable means of long-term life support. Now, they give me a glimpse of the beginning of time and the power of reason. I think that I may have been permitted a shimmering glimmer of sense of the mystery of the atom. I will find myself lost in thought in the strangest of places, if sometimes not the safest of places, such as two weeks ago, when I was driving to work, paying my usual amount of attention to the road, and I noticed the sun. It was a clear day, with a sky so blue that it hurt my eyes to look at it, and momentarily, I found myself wondering why there were shadows.

In 400 BC, nearly two hundred years before a man pounded a stake into the ground and measured the circumference of the earth, another conceived of the atom as the basic structure of matter. The first man, from 400 BC, was a Greek, known as Democritus. He was from Thrace in northern Greece and believed that everything was composed of atoms which were indivisible, separated by space, and always in motion. In 250 BC the second man, Eratosthenes of Alexandria of ancient Egypt, measured the circumference of the earth at 39,250 km, which was accurate to within 2 percent.

A contemporary of Democritus, in time but not in place, being separated by the land mass of Greece and the Ionian Sea, on the east side of Italy, was Empedocles of Sicily, who thought he was a god. To prove this point, he leapt into the volcanic crater of Etna and was never heard from again. Empedocles is credited with proposing the four basic elements: earth, air, fire and water, from which everything was made. Prior to him, the men of science thought that either fire, water, or air, alone, was the primordial element from which all else was made.

A century after Democritus and a century before Eratosthenes, in 360 BC, finds us back across the Ionian Sea, north of the city walls of ancient Athens in a sacred grove of olive trees, dedicated to Athena, the goddess of wisdom. It was named Akademia, after a Greek war hero, and was spared by the Spartans, out of respect, during the five invasions of Attica over the course of the thirty-year Peloponnesian War. This sacred grove of olive trees, which was connected to Athens by a road, lined with the graves of Athenian soldiers and within a walk of the Saronic Gulf of the Sea of Crete, became the site of Plato's Academy.

In 360 BC a young man was taught by the teacher, who himself was a student of Socrates. They sat in the shade of an olive tree under a sunlit sky so blue that it hurt their eyes to look at it. Together, they had a discourse of the four elements. Later, the young man, known by the name of Aristotle, proposed a fifth element, quintessence, of which the heavenly bodies are composed. He went on to define an element as something that cannot decompose or be divided any further.

Socrates taught Plato, who taught Aristotle, who taught Alexander the Great. Alexander the Great, son of Philip of Macedonia, went on to conquer the known world at the time. The city named after him, Alexandria, the setting of Antony and Cleopatra, *was the home of Eratosthenes, a man who pounded a stake into the ground on a sunny day, under a blue sky, and measured the circumference of the earth to within 2 percent.*

The periodic table is the chart containing all of the elements which, you might recall from science class, looked kind of like a calendar. In Democritus' day, had it been invented, the periodic table would have contained four squares, for the four elements of earth, air, fire, and water. The periodic table of 2006 contains 117 squares for all the elements, 94 of these naturally occurring on earth. Everything is made of these 94 elements, including, of course, us. The term atom *is derived from the Greek word* atomos *meaning* uncuttable, *which is incorrect, as an atom is composed of subatomic particles: electrons, protons, and neutrons. Protons and neutrons are composed of quarks, of which there are six different kinds. So atoms make up molecules that make up compounds that form cellular elements that compose our organ systems that become us, as well as everything that is not us.*

What most people don't realize is that the atom is mostly space—99.999 percent space. There is much more space within the atomic structure than ever was conceived of by Democritus in 420 BC. I suspect that his concept of space may have had more to do with the space between atoms rather than the space within the atom.

The planetary model of a sun-like nucleus surrounded by planet-like electrons gives a false sense of proximity. To put the capaciousness of the atom in perspective, consider a football stadium—Lambeau Field. Now, imagine a marble centered on the fifty-yard line of the frozen tundra, and a speck of dust swirling around in the bowl of the stadium and up to three blocks into the surrounding neighborhood. This space would be representative of a hydrogen atom with one proton, comprising the nucleus (marble) and one electron (speck of dust) in orbit around the nucleus. To quantize this further, the size of the three-dimensional orbit of the electron, around the nucleus, is up to 100,000 times the size of the nucleus itself; and the size of the electron is $\frac{1}{1,800}^{th}$ that of the nucleus.

So I was wondering, if everything is mostly space, why don't photons, which are the mass-less subatomic particles of light radiating from the sun at 186,000 miles per second, simply pass through all this space to illuminate a shadow-less world? *Hmmmm...* I glanced heavenward, much as Archimedes must have done while soaking in his bath just before he realized the principle of displacement and how he could tell if the king's crown was made of solid gold or not—*it was not*. Although handicapped by a markedly diminished intellect, relative to Archimedes, I did have the benefit of several hundred years of scientific evolution and fourteen years of post-graduate education heavily weighted in the sciences. Combined with my matured reading habits, this was sufficient such that I was able to arrive at a plausible explanation before swerving across the center line.

There are four fundamental forces in all the universe. Of these, only two are readily apparent. The fundamental force we will focus on first is the one that is found between the positively charged proton(s) in the atomic nucleus and the negatively charged electron(s) out in orbit—this is the electromagnetic force. It is this energy field that repels the orbits of other electrons from other atoms. If the space of an atom were invaded by electrons of other atoms, then the atom would lose its structural integrity and would no longer be what it once was. A component of this force that you can actually feel is that which you experience in trying to push the similar poles of two magnets together. The closer they get, the stronger the force, and if the magnets were big enough you wouldn't be able to push them together at all. It is this electrical energy, between the proton(s) in the nucleus and the electron(s) in orbit, which is responsible for solidity. It is this electrical energy, found in the chemical bonds of food, which accounts for the caloric content of our daily diet.

In high school we were most likely taught Niels Bohr's model of the atom, in which the atom looks like a planetary system, which it really isn't. The orbiting electrons are represented by plump, spherical planets, which they really aren't. And the nucleus, in the middle of the symmetrically defined orbits of the planetary electrons, is represented by an even plumper, spherical "sun," which isn't nearly as straightforward as it looks.

If an atom doesn't look like the diagram, what exactly is it?

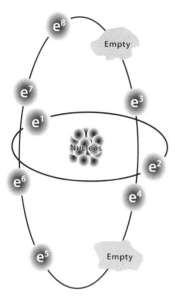

Diagram of oxygen
The two orbital shells can hold a maximum of two electrons in the inner shell and eight electrons in the outer shell. Because there are only six electrons in the outer shell, which can hold up to eight, there are two "empty" spaces that can share electrons of another atom.

For example, if oxygen shares its two empty spaces with two hydrogen atoms, the molecular formula is H_2O (see page 154).

First of all, think of the nucleus. The nucleus is the center of an atom and is made of subatomic particles that are all very mysterious. The basic ones that we know about are neutrons and protons. The neutrons have no electrical charge and the protons have a positive charge. It is the positive charge of the proton in the nucleus that attracts the negative charge of the electron. This electrical attraction is what keeps the electron in its orbit around the nucleus. It is this very important electrical attraction that makes the atom, and therefore the elements, and therefore us, possible.

Now, imagine all the particles of the nucleus (neutrons and protons) clumped together by an immensely powerful force that is one hundred times stronger than the electromagnetic force. This force is the second of the four fundamental forces of the universe and is known as the strong nuclear force. Without the strong nuclear force there would be no nuclei for the simple reason that the protons' natural tendency is to repel one another because of their like, positive charges. And if there were no nuclei, then there would be no atoms, and if there were no atoms...

Surrounding this conglomeration of protons and neutrons called a nucleus are minute particles—electrons—spinning at speeds approaching the speed of light. The electrons (negative charge) are attracted to the equal number of protons (positive charge) by the same electrical force that we witness with every flip of a switch.

The electrons inhabit a spherical space up to 100,000 times the size of the nucleus at its center, and are moving so fast that it seems as though they are everywhere at once, as if each nucleus is surrounded by a cloud of electrons. This capacious space, relative to the size of the nucleus, is organized into spherical (orbital) shells and each shell can contain a limited number of electrons: two in the first shell, eight in the second shell and more are allowed with more shells. Each electron occupies a specific, nonidentical space within its orbital shell, and although the electron moves at speeds approaching the speed of light, appearing as a cloud rather than a series of individual points, it is a very specific cloud—one that is unique to each lone electron.

The reason you don't fall through the chair you're sitting on is because it is impossible for the electrons occupying specific spaces in the space of your butt to invade the specific spaces of the electrons of the wood, cushion, nylon webbing, toilet seat, or whatever firm surface it is that is keeping you from plunging towards the center of the earth. It is this electromagnetic force, like the attraction between the six electrons and six protons of the carbon atom, which represents the chemical energy of the food we eat that is measured with the unit of energy of the calorie. It is this electromagnetic energy that we consume that is transferred to our biological energy systems through the process of metabolism that sustains our lives. It is this elec-

tromagnetic energy that if consumed in excess is converted to stored energy in the form of fat. In our Herculean efforts to comprehend the why and the how of positive thought and weight loss, not to mention quantum theory, we need to understand that when we are losing weight, we are losing mostly space.

Okay. So electricity keeps my hand from reaching through a steel door. What about photons, which are particles of light that have zero charge and zero mass— why don't they "shine" through solid objects, not creating shadows? A semi blew past me, wanting to make the light at the intersection I was approaching. Its jet stream pushed me towards the shoulder as I thought, *Maybe some photons do shine through, but most would be absorbed by the matter encountered, imparting energy to that matter.* I remembered the heat of asphalt on bare feet at Murphy Park on a sunny day, and the hot seat of a car parked in the sun—that heat represents the energy of photons of the sun, from the fusion (coming together) of four atoms of hydrogen into one atom of helium, 94 million miles away.

I thought about photons being absorbed, deflected and reflected, and as I flipped the signal lever down, to turn right towards the hospital, I had another thought. Suppose there is an object of variable thickness, such as a round pole, then the edges of the shadow should be less intense or maybe a little blurry because of more photons *shining through* the thinnest part of the pole. As I approached the entry of Door County Memorial Hospital, I conveniently encountered a few round metal poles and noted that, indeed, the edges were blurry, for whichever reason. I stood there on that crisp, bright day in February, looking at that shadow of a pole and thought, *I should probably go swimming today.*

⧓

It wouldn't be fair to leave this section without defining the four fundamental forces more completely and putting them in perspective as, after all, this book is a book of energy: of understanding energy, of eating energy, of storing energy, and of expending energy. Thus far, we have touched upon the strong nuclear force that hints at the massiveness of nuclear energy, and the electromagnetic force that powers our computers and is the ultimate source of the chemical energy of the food and fuels of our daily lives.

The four fundamental forces of the universe

1. Electromagnetic force
2. Strong nuclear force
3. Weak nuclear force
4. Gravity

Why is the nuclear force so perfectly strong? It has to be. A hydrogen atom only has one proton, but a carbon atom has six. Remember that like charges repel (the two similar poles of a magnet). The six protons of the carbon atom don't want to be clumped together in an infinitesimally small space. The only way they can be held so tightly is by the strong nuclear force. If the strong nuclear force was just a tiny bit different either way—more or less— our universe wouldn't exist. This is only one of the "Goldilocks" conditions of our third planet from the sun that makes life possible in our universe. This exact relative strength of the strong nuclear force is only one small but significant part of the cosmic porridge where things are just right, not too hot and not too cold, in which life, in which our lives become possible.

The weak nuclear force is only observed at the nuclear level and is related to radioactive decay. This is not commonly observed in everyday life and consequently will receive only this brief mention.

The final and by far the weakest of the fundamental forces is the force of Newtonian fame, that being *gravity*. If gravity is assigned a relative strength of one, the relative strength of the strong nuclear force is about one hundred thousand million, billion, billion, billion or 10^{38}. Clearly, gravity is not insignificant despite its relative weakness. It is responsible for keeping our planet in orbit around the sun and our feet upon the earth. It is as big as the atomic scale is small. The gravitational force is exerted over hundreds of thousands of miles, as opposed to the microscopic scale of the atom with a nuclear size of about 10^{-14} meters. It is Sir Isaac's elucidation of gravity and the natural laws of classical physics that have graced the age of man, launching humankind from the very face of the earth.

If gravity is at one end of the spectrum of the four fundamental forces, then the strong nuclear force is at the opposite end, in terms of distance and relative strength, with about forty powers of ten between them (a 1 followed by 40 zeros). This strong nuclear force is in us, in the water, in the food we eat, the oil we burn—wherever there are atoms, which is obviously everywhere. In belaboring the weakness of gravity when compared to the strong nuclear force, I should note that it's not that gravity is so weak; rather, it's that the strong nuclear force is so magnificently strong.

Richard Feynman gave a physics lecture in the sixties and illustrated the power inherent within the atomic nucleus: "…the energy that can be obtained from 10 quarts of water per second is equal to all of the electrical power generated in the United States. With 150 gallons of running water a minute, you have enough fuel to supply all the energy which is used in the United States today!"[27]

Newton told us that for every action there is an opposite and equal reaction—his third law of motion. With this in mind, consider the complex chain of events resulting in the unleashing of the strong nuclear force in the detonation of Little Boy.

Action: Two chunks of uranium-235, weighing a total of sixty-four kilograms, drop from the belly of the Enola Gay at 8:15:19, August 6th, 1944. Forty-three seconds later, 1,900 feet above ground and 550 feet southeast of the target of Aioi Bridge, the two pieces of metal, from opposite ends of a gun tube, are smashed together by the force of a chemical explosive charge.

Reaction: Only a small fraction of a pound of the uranium is converted into energy with the chain reaction release of the strong nuclear force. Cloudless skies, a quiet early morning of eighty degrees and 80 percent humidity becomes, in one tenth of a second, a fiery cauldron of dry black heat with a temperature of 5,400 degrees at the hypocenter, due to the 12.5-kiloton explosion (25 million pounds of TNT) from the release of energy from a small pebble of uranium of a weight barely perceptible in the palm of your hand.[28] If there were ever any doubt that the age of man had arrived, there was no more, as the intellectual descendants of Democritus, Eratosthenes and Aristotle had created on earth, from a lump of warm metal, the very energy of the sun.

I appreciate the fact that this is unlike any diet book you've ever read. It isn't, really, a diet book. I want it to be much more than that. My intent is for this to be a life-changing book of which weight loss is only a side effect. Our progression requires building blocks and we have a few more ahead of us, so please allow me to briefly summarize the scientific aspects of the first half of the first pillar of emotional health.

The universe is composed of organic (implying biological life) and inorganic (like a rock) material. The material is composed of compounds that are composed of molecules that are composed of atoms that are composed of subatomic particles (neutrons, electrons, protons, etc.) that are composed of quarks that are composed of ???

Our solidity is due to the electrical energy of atoms in constant motion, which is illustrated by a gross simplification of Einstein's famous equation, $E = mc^2$, defining energy as mass in motion—energy is equivalent to mass. Our physical bodies are more than 99 percent space holding vast amounts of energy, most of which is safely locked away in our atomic nuclei.

What does this mean for me, for us, and can we modify this in any way? A comprehension of our composition is, I think, liberating, and an important part of our continuing journey. Our newfound awareness hints at the malleability of our physical form and the power within ourselves to change it, which is the continuing focus of pillars two and three.

The balance of our time in the first pillar will focus on the background and means of effecting a positive change in our lives, both emotional and physical. This will require a few more building blocks and so let us return to the universe and, specifically, the uncertainty and probability of life.

My goal in trying to turn all of you into theoretical nuclear physicists is twofold.

Firstly, I feel that a comprehension of our physical form is vital in learning how to harness the power of positive energy and optimism. Secondly, it is crucial in understanding the meaning of the calorie and the energy density of food and then applying that knowledge to the pursuit of a healthy lifestyle and long-term weight loss.

Throughout history great minds have been visited upon this earth and this is how we started this section, with Eratosthenes, Democritus and Aristotle. Now, twenty-five hundred years later there came another collection of great minds, clustered around the time before the first of two world wars: a collection of men with names like Max Planck, Niels Bohr, Werner Heisenberg, Erwin Schrödinger, Albert Einstein, and yes, Ernest Hemingway, and I could go on. It is absolutely amazing, this collection of intellect at this time in our history. And now it is time to take what we have just learned about atomic theory and carry it a bit further.

chapter eight

The quantum mechanics
of a better life

I F ONLY I COULD say *don't worry, be happy* and it would be so. If only I could fill you with a ream of feel-good stories, such that the draft of positive afterglow would suffuse your being, delivering success and happiness into your everyday life.

I can't do that; however, I can do this: I can exert a subtle or a not so subtle force against you with words and ideas that will cause a reaction that results in another, such that you'll experience your own chain reaction that just might positively alter the course of your life. *Do you feel me yet? Do you hear me now?*

Your reaction will involve more than that clutch in your throat from reading soulful stories. I'm asking you to do more. Your reaction will require an active participation with the universe, in a manner of speaking. There are hundreds of self-help books focusing on positive thinking and imagery and they make valid points, but I haven't come across one that explained *why or how* to my satisfaction.

I read this best seller of a book in Target one afternoon over the course of an hour, because it was short, and that's how long it took my wife to walk up and down every aisle, putting things in the cart that she didn't know she needed until she got there. This was before my reading habits matured, so I didn't buy the book at the time, as it was not fiction. It spoke of positive thinking and *laws of attraction*. It was nicely packaged, with the suggestion that the key to happiness and success really was a long-lost secret from thousands of years ago that lay buried underground in a tomb somewhere in the Mideast—Egypt, I think, because I saw a picture of a pyramid. I ran across a planetary model of the atom and some mention was made of energy and vibration, as I recollect. I remember being disappointed, because I wanted to believe in some form of empowerment with which to improve my life; but it seemed too superficial to me, like all I had to do was think about being happy and successful and eventually it would magically come true. There was no explanation, really, of *how*, and certainly not of *why* that made any sense to me.

With our recently acquired knowledge of the atom and subatomic particles, we are able to delve deeper into quantum physics to better understand the role of energy in our lives and what control we might exert over it. There are two ways in which we could do this: either with a lot of math and a little language, or a whole lot of language and zero math. As a matter of convenience, I will presume that my broader audience would prefer the latter method, because I am ill-prepared to present the former.

Ill-prepared through no fault of intellect I would hope; rather, in the spirit of not blaming self, I would instead assign fault to Sister Carol, since she is long deceased and not around to defend herself. I only assume that she has shed these mortal coils as she was absolutely ancient thirty-five years ago when our paths first crossed, in my freshman algebra class. It may very well be that she'll show up on my front doorstep one day, dressed in her familiar black, like an avenging ninja angel of retribution, to lay a curse on my soul for what I am about to reveal.

Well into her seventies at the time of our first meeting, she weighed no more than ninety pounds and was almost two feet taller than a yardstick, in a curvilinear sort of way. I couldn't tell you much more than that, because all I ever saw of her was her face and the tips of matte black shoes. Everything else was flowing black robes that swallowed up a stooped, shriveled, humanoid form—and I wasn't even sure of that. The starched white habit she wore pinched her face, which only accentuated her androgynous features and created a circumferential wrinkle around her face, lending the appearance of an oval picture frame of dry flaking skin.

I could not associate the concept of "hair" with Sr. Carol, as I never saw any on her hands or peeking out from under her habit; and I recall one day in class when she happened to pass a heat register. A warm blast of air floated the black veil of her habit heavenwards. As I was sitting down, it was almost like a reflex for me to glance up and under, in curious anticipation of a forbidden world; and although I was seated right next to that very same register, blasting dry ninety-degree air, an icy shiver of dread raced through my body at the shaded sight of her nearly bald head.

Her complexion held an ever so subtle tint of lime in the morning sun; and her chapped lips suggested a perpetual state of dehydration, as though she had just spent forty days and forty nights in the desert. In short, I was never convinced that Sister Carol was one of us; and thought instead that she may have been an alien life-form from an arid planet inhabited by little green men.

I asked only one question during my freshman algebra class, and that was in the second week. We had just begun instruction on the quadratic equation ($ax^2 + bx + c = 0$) and I couldn't quite grasp the concept.

I raised my hand and asked, "Sister Carol, does the sum of all the coefficients *always* equal zero?"

Expectant waiting ensued. Not many questions had been asked as of yet in freshman algebra.

"We-ell..." she said. A pregnant pause ensued. I imagined frayed synaptic connections, crackling and hissing from the friction of thought. "...Because!" she snarled, swiveling her head around, like Linda Blair in *The Exorcist*, sans projectile green vomit. Her face was scrunched up in a heavy scowl and her squinty eyes, inflamed from a chronic conjunctivitis, speared me with a disgruntled gaze communicating to the class the general impression of—*what a stupid question.*

My self-esteem collapsed, being overburdened as it was from a severe acne problem, the tail end of my "husky phase," and the lack of any athletic grace whatsoever. From that day forward, the mere mention of any mathematical formula with an "*x*" in it would trigger an instant state of panic.

⌗

Sister Hugo was as big as Sister Carol was small. I know for sure that Sister Hugo is gone because I heard of it through the Catholic grapevine during medical school. She died of heart disease and complications of diabetes, no doubt secondary to her markedly elevated BMI. Sister Hugo didn't share Sister Carol's sense of austerity in matters of dress. I could see that Sister Hugo had legs, thick ones, covered with opaque tan support hose and shod in the standard black-leather sister-shoe; and, rather than the habit of Sister Carol, which was more like the helmet of a dark lady-knight of God, she wore a black veil-like thing bobby-pinned to the back of her head, which suggested more of a nurse from hell than a bride of Christ.

Sister Hugo was my sophomore English teacher. She liked boys, I think because she viewed girls as inherently wicked, probably because of that story about the apple (*or was it an apricot*) in the garden. Most of us blessed with the Y chromosome and half a brain got A's in her class. I must have a whole brain because I got A+'s. The double XX did less well, unless exceptionally bright. One day it was my turn to give an audio-visual presentation. I delivered a speech about scuba diving and the coral reef, accompanied by a slide show. Halfway through my presentation I heard sniffling behind me. As my final slide of a sunset over the Caribbean dropped into the tray, suppressed emotional breathing gave way to breast-heaving, sinus-clearing sobs. Thinking that something terrible must have happened, I turned around to see Sister Hugo's flushed fleshy cheeks stained with tears.

"It's SO BEAUTIFUL," she gasped. Her hands were clasped together in front of her, as though she had just swallowed the body of Christ. "Isn't it, class?"

I didn't hear anyone else crying; but I could see another A+ looming in my immediate future.

God bless both the sisters' respective energies, loosed upon the universe, but perhaps Sister Hugo's a little more because she gave me language, and it is with language that I will address certain aspects of quantum theory: the uncertainty principle, the double-slit lamp experiment, Schrödinger's cat, and the many worlds theory, which will be helpful to us in our journey towards enlightenment.

The uncertainty principle

Werner Heisenberg was a young physicist who joined Niels Bohr as a research assistant in Copenhagen during the decade of the twenties. Heisenberg was trying to address the question of how to measure the location of an electron around a nucleus. He demonstrated that you could measure the position and the momentum of a particle (electron) but the more accurately you determined one, the less accurately you knew the other. Perhaps it would be more accurate to say that no matter how hard he tried, Heisenberg couldn't measure the exact position and the exact momentum of an electron *at the same time.* As soon as he measured the exact position, it became impossible to define the precise momentum. And as soon as he measured the precise momentum, it became impossible to measure the exact position. You might say that an electron would most likely be *here,* but could also show up *over there.* It was, and still is, impossible to know both an electron's exact position and where it is going *at the same time.* Heisenberg mathematically represented the uncertainty principle with the following formula:

$$\Delta x \Delta p \geq \frac{\hbar}{2}$$

where Δx represents the *change in position,* Δp represents the *change in momentum* (mass × velocity), and $\hbar$

represents *Planck's constant*, which is a very small number, in the neighborhood of 10^{-34}—that is zero point thirty-three zeros followed by a one—a billion trillion trillionth of a meter.

Because of the size scale (10^{-34}), one might argue that the uncertainty principle is of questionable significance from an observational standpoint; nonetheless, the very existence of uncertainty, which Heisenberg scientifically proved, unleashed subsequent years of debate arguing for and against it. The problem created by the discovery of uncertainty, and of quantum theory in general, is that it was not consistent with Newton's laws of motion and Einstein's general relativity. Theoretically, using the laws of classical physics, one should be able to measure the mass, force, and distances traveled of a particle and thereby predict the exact position of each particle in the universe and where it was going, which in effect would be *predicting the future*. This gap between quantum theory and classical physics still exists today, awaiting a "Grand Unification Theory," or "Theory of Everything."

One interpretation of the quantum mechanics of the uncertainty principle is called the Copenhagen interpretation because it arose at that point in history in which much of the collective thought evolved in that part of Europe, Copenhagen being the home of Niels Bohr. This interpretation states that the position and momentum of every particle are defined by a special type of a mathematical formula called a wave function. It's not that the electron *is* everywhere at the same time; rather, it *could be everywhere* at the same time. The wave function will yield *a probability of position,* but the exact position of a particle is only revealed when the particle is observed. So, although you can measure the exact position of an electron, or a photon for that matter, it is impossible to know by which path it arrived or where, exactly, it came from. You may be tempted to think that *yeah, but that was in the 1920s;* however, even with the infinitely more precise measurements that are available today, the Copenhagen interpretation still holds, uncertainty exists, and Heisenberg's uncertainty principle has not been disproven.

Double-slit lamp experiment

There is one experiment that epitomizes the mystery of quantum mechanics that has been performed through-out the years in ever more elegant fashions. It has yielded the same result every time—an unexplainable result illuminating the unknown and uncertainty that is interwoven into the fabric of our existence. The double-slit experiment originally involved the projection of light (photons) against a barrier with two vertical slits. On the other side of the barrier was a detection screen on which the resulting pattern of light could be observed. The experiment was performed for the first time in 1801 by Thomas Young using sunlight shining through a pinhole into a darkened room. The result proved unequivocally that light behaved as a wave, like ripples on the smooth surface of a pond that result from a thrown stone. Light was not a particle, like a bullet from a gun existing only along a specific trajectory; no, light traveled in waves, existing in many different places along the wave front *at the same time.*

A little over one hundred years later, in 1905, Einstein published the mathematical definition of the *photoelec-tric effect*, which proved that *no, light is not a wave*, but rather, it is a particle of "light quanta," now called a *pho-*

ton. It was for this work that Einstein was specifically noted in his 1921 Nobel Prize, not for his theory of relativity. Because of his work on the photoelectric effect at the turn of the century and Young's experiment a hundred years earlier, there was at that point in history scientific proof that light behaved both as a wave and as a particle. It behaved as a wave for Thomas Young in 1801, seventy-eight years before the invention of the lightbulb, and it behaved as a particle for Albert Einstein in 1905, forty years before the Trinity test (first nuclear explosion).

In the year of my birth, 1961, a man by the name of Claus Jönsson repeated the double-slit experiment again, this time not with light, but with electrons that were fired one at a time, just like BB's from a gun. This experiment was voted "the most beautiful experiment" by *Physics World* readers in 2002. Apart from the electrons, which represented actual mass, as opposed to the mass-less photons of Thomas Young, everything else was much the same; there were two apertures (slits) that the electrons had to travel through, and there was the detector screen on the other side which revealed the pattern of their landing.

Since all the great minds, past and present, in the universe of physics could not explain the double-slit experiment, I think that the easiest thing for me to do at this point is to simply show you the schematic representations of what you might think the outcome should be, and then what the actual outcome is, and then you can be as puzzled as were Einstein, Feynman and everyone else.

First, let's do the double-slit experiment with light. We'll shine a light through a double-slit screen and you might think that it would look something like this:

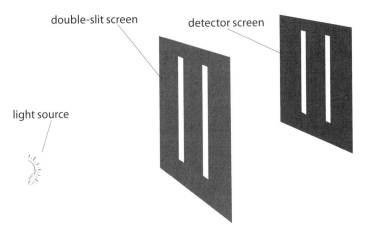

Intuitive outcome with both slits open

The actual outcome, the outcome that Thomas Young observed more than two hundred years ago, looked more like this.

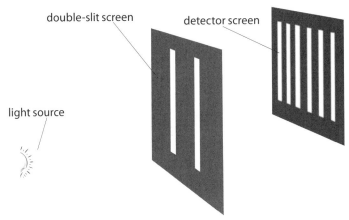

Actual outcome with both slits open

So, what does this mean? Well, at Mr. Young's point in history, this was proof that light behaved as a wave. If light were a particle, existing at only one point in time and traveling in a specific trajectory, like a bullet, the outcome would be like our intuitive outcome in the first diagram because each particle of light would strike the screen immediately behind each open slit.

But, when light travels as a wave, existing everywhere along the wave front at once, then the outcome is that of what is observed in the second diagram because, as the wave of light hits the two slits, it is split into two waves, which then *interfere* with each other. And in fact, this observable pattern is called an *interference pattern*, which is typical wave behavior, like the ripples from one tossed pebble interfering with those of another.

So what, you might think. Big deal; but, remember. Einstein proved that light was a *quanta*, a particle that we now call a photon. When Claus Jönsson repeated the experiment 160 years later with electrons, which are obviously particles of mass, he discovered that *the electrons behaved like waves as well.* Remember, in this experiment the electrons were fired one at a time, with each individual electron being detected on the screen after traveling through one slit or the other. Since we already know that electrons are particles, you would expect the outcome to be something like the illustration at the top of the next page.

What Claus Jönsson observed on one particular and interesting day in the same year that I was pulled headfirst from my mother's birth canal was more like the illustration at the bottom of the next page.

He saw a seemingly random pattern of electrons on the screen; so, he waited longer. After a few more

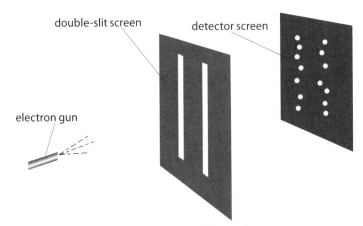

Intuitive outcome with both slits open

million electrons impacted the screen, one after the other, and all the little white dots became somewhat confluent, what he then saw is shown at the top of the next page.

What Claus Jönsson saw was the interference pattern, even though the electrons were fired one at a time. Now, if a million billion photons or electrons are released at

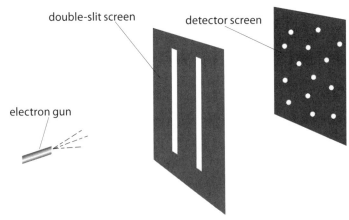

Actual outcome with both slits open

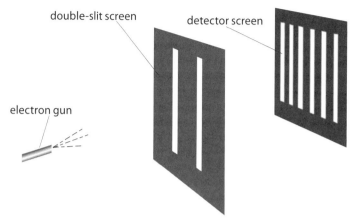

Actual outcome with both slits open after several million electrons

one time, it is easy to imagine them all interfering with one another, but, how can there be interference if the particles are released *one at a time? Hmmm, that's the sticky-wicky.* If the electron travels like a wave, doesn't that mean that it has to go through both slits *at the same time,* just like a wave of light or water does? Theoretically, the seeming reality is that the electron travels every possible path in order to arrive at its exact particle-spot on the detector screen, which would look something like the illustration at the top of the next page.

Kind of spooky. Well then, think about this—the experiment has been performed with a little detector off to the side to see which slit the electrons, fired one at time, go through—the experimenter peeks between the double-slit screen and the detector plate. *What do you think happens?* You do find out which slit each electron goes through, but then, instead of the alternating bands of the interference pattern, you see only the two vertical bands of particle behavior. The wave behavior collapses and the electrons behave like particles and the

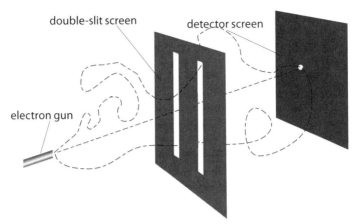

The lone electron travels every possible path.

interference pattern disappears. As soon as the detector is removed, the interference pattern reappears, as illustrated previously.

The interference pattern is observed only if no one is looking. It is as though the electron knows when someone is watching. It is as though the electron knows in advance what you are doing. This experiment has been performed numerous times, with different particles of matter and light, and the result is always the same—spooky and unexplainable.

You may be wondering—*what the hell is he talking about? What has this to do with anything about weight loss?* To which I would reply:

"Please, dear reader, do not grow impatient.

"Seek not to know the answer; rather, to understand the question."

The point of the double-slit experiment is that it represents a stunningly beautiful physical proof of uncertainty. It is what it is. It tells us that nothing is meant to be. Nothing is predetermined or foreordained. No one is meant to be obese or unhappy all the days of their lives—these unfortunate situations of life represent outcomes, not destinies. This will be developed further within the next few pages, and as a few more grains of sand drop, from the upper bowl of the hourglass to its bottom, the proof of happiness will be revealed.

Schrödinger's cat

I think that it is safe to say that we now all have a common understanding of the existence, or lack thereof, of the electron. Remember that we are talking of course about basic particles of matter. This is the stuff of the food we eat, the stuff of which our bodies and mind are made. We are nothing more than atoms made of space, electrons and the other particles of matter, all driven by the electricity of our thought.

Now, we have started in 400 BC with Democritus and have just spent time with Jönsson of modern day, but let us go back now to the time of Schrödinger, Einstein, Heisenberg and Bohr. A time in the world of physics, before the advent of electron guns, particle accelerators and electron microscopes, when all these great minds wrestled with the concept of uncertainty using only the electricity of thought.

There was a popular *thought* experiment at the time which still generates endless discussions today. It is known as *Schrödinger's cat.* Erwin Schrödinger was a proponent of the Copenhagen interpretation, which Einstein did not embrace enthusiastically because of the implied uncertainty. In discussions with Einstein, Schrödinger posited a thought experiment having to do with a cat in a box. I would hazard a guess that Erwin had a dog, because I'm thinking he was not particularly fond of cats, as you will see.

Imagine a cat in a box which no one can see inside of, and just like Las Vegas, whatever happens in the box stays in the box. In this box with the cat is a lead container that has inside of it some radioactive material that may or may not decay. The lead container has a shutter that will open just long enough to allow a fifty percent probability that decay will occur. If decay occurs, then a particle is released that triggers a hammer to fall. When the hammer falls, it breaks a glass vial, which releases a poison that causes the death of the cat.

For an observer outside of the box, after the shutter has deployed, is the cat alive or dead? If I were a follower of the Copenhagen interpretation, I would suggest that the cat is neither. It is half dead and half alive. It will only become one or the other after opening the box—it is only real if it is observed. Recall the electrons in the double slit? In accordance with the Copenhagen interpretation, the interference pattern is a representation of a *probability* of where the electron could land. All the potential pathways of the electrons are only possibilities based on probability and, like the half-alive/half-dead cat, do not exist until they are observed. The only real thing is that which is observed; namely, that little white dot of an electron that shows up on the screen here or there and, in this case, a live cat or a dead one.

Schrödinger was the first to write down the wave equation at the center of the Copenhagen interpretation, which is a mathematical equation that gives a probability distribution of finding a particle at a certain position. The values obtained by the equation are consistent with the natural laws of known physics, one of its tests being the measurement of the energy levels of the hydrogen atom.[29]

There is yet another interpretation of quantum mechanics born out of a doctoral thesis by Hugh Everett in 1957 and later developed further by Bryce DeWitt, who called this theory the many worlds interpretation. If I were a follower of the many worlds interpretation I would submit that the cat is both alive and dead. When I open the box and Tinkerbelle jumps into my arms to give my cheek a scratchy lick—at that very moment, in an alternate reality branching off from my current reality, there is another "me" opening another door to another box with a dead Tinkerbelle in it. In the many worlds theory the electron *does* travel every possible path; it's just that we are only aware of the one path in our reality. Everything is real. There are infinitely branching alternate realities that are constantly bifurcating from our current reality such that our reality runs in parallel with every other reality accounting for every possible path or outcome. How do I know if I'm in the *real* reality, or one of the alternate ones? *Hmmm, another sticky-wicky.* I suppose it is a matter of relativity. From the frame of reference of inhabitants of another reality, like maybe the one in which I am president and everything is perfect, I suppose the "me" writing this now would be in an alternate reality.

Sounds crazy—I know—but that's quantum theory for you. These are two of the chief competing theories of our existence, today, in modern times, each theory having a mathematical background to support it. This is what the professionals actually think, although I should say that the majority subscribe to the Copenhagen interpretation.

Quantum theory is almost like religion in that it requires a leap of faith, a suspension of belief, to believe in something that we cannot see, something that is not consistent with reality as we know it. At one end of the spectrum are the disciples of the Copenhagen interpretation, who believe only in what is observed—the cat is half alive and half dead, only becoming one or the other when it is observed; and the electron travels a probability of paths, which collapses to one path only when it is observed. At the other end of the spectrum are the disciples of the many worlds interpretation, who believe in alternate realities, in which everything is real; there is both a live cat and a dead cat, and the electron travels every path, but we only see the one cat or the one electron in our own reality/universe.

In the world of quantum theory, much is possible. It is possible for an electron and its anti-particle, which is called a positron, to transiently manifest from two energized photons in a process called pair production. The brief existence of the positron is only as long as it takes for it to meet an electron, in which case the positive charge of the positron is annihilated by the negative charge of the electron, with the result being, again, two highly energized photons with zero mass and zero charge. This represents the appearance of mass and electrical charge out of nothing with the abrupt conversion back to nothingness. *Was it really there?* Yes, the annihilation of the positron with an electron is the subatomic reality behind the positron emission tomography (PET scan) that is widely used every day for the detection of cancer.

In the world of quantum theory there is a mathematical formula that yields a probability of me hiking across the far side of the moon. There is a parallel universe in which everyone speaks German. And, there is the fourth dimension of time, where forwards and backwards for subatomic particles are probably much the same as the spatial dimensions of right and left or up and down are to us.

On the quantum scale of time the same thing looks completely different depending upon whether you are approaching it antegrade (forward moving) or retrograde (backward moving) on the time scale. Are the electron and positron becoming photons or are the photons becoming an electron and a positron? *Well, that depends;* in fact, the equivalent of the positron, which has the same mass as the electron and the exact opposite charge, is that of an electron *traveling back in time.*

At the macro level, where we live and breathe, on a scale greater than or equal to a millimeter (10^{-3}) and at speeds less than the speed of sound (340 meters/sec), quantum mechanical action is as a smooth edge stretching, unbroken, as far as the eye can see. Its effects are so far below our powers of observation that they are invisible to us. Conversely, from the quantum standpoint of an electron, which exists on the Planck scale of 10^{-34} m and at speeds of light, our macro world is nearly standing still, frozen in time. *There is no edge.*

In our universe, it is thought that the net balance of positive and negative energy is very close to zero, if not equal to zero. By this I mean to say that all of the positive energy, which is represented by the mass of the universe, is balanced by the negative energy of gravity. The energy of gravity is considered negative because lifting something up *against gravity* represents positive energy. Theoretically, to some, the universe, which has been expanding since the Big Bang, exists only on borrowed time, eventually reaching a point, like a stretched-out rubber band, from which it will contract. The contracting universe will then ultimately collapse, annihilating itself like the electron-positron pair, which exists for only a fraction of a fraction of a second—a time so brief that it may as well never have happened—*but it did.*[30]

Application of quantum mechanics

My purpose in dragging you through these aspects of quantum theory is to offer you a glimpse of the reality of what we are—contained collections of energy, of primarily space, made solid by fundamental forces and natural law—possessing awareness of our own existence.

It doesn't matter if you subscribe to the Copenhagen interpretation or the many worlds theory, or neither, for that matter. The reality is that there is a natural law of uncertainty. The universe is therefore nondeterministic. Outcomes cannot be known. The only *known* is a probability of a certain outcome. The inference is that I can influence the probability of an outcome by my thoughts and actions.

There are an infinite number of pathways branching out in front of me. Either each pathway represents only a probability, *only one* of which I will observe, thereby making it real; or an infinite number of pathways exist and are chosen by an infinite number of alternate existences *of me* in alternate universes, of which I can only be aware of the one that I inhabit.

> *The reality of uncertainty is that I can choose*
>   *or influence a probability; or*
> *The reality of uncertainty is that I can choose*
>   *or influence an "alternate" universe.*

I have mentioned both positive and negative energy in the physical sense, in regard to the total mass and amount of gravity of the universe. I also have mentioned positive energy in the metaphysical sense, in regard to the power of positive thought and optimism. There is also the matter of negative energy in the metaphysical sense, which pertains to negative thinking and pessimism.

Often in life we will find ourselves observing a probability or living a reality not of our choosing, but which we must react to. This reality may be a negative one, such as the loss of a loved one or the diagnosis of a serious illness, which is a representation of the tragedy of life that we discussed earlier—that necessary component of our human condition. At that specific point in time, there are multiple probabilities/realities before us. We are free to choose a positive one or a negative one. We will move forward in time in a positive direction, or a negative one, based upon our choice.

Please don't think that I am discounting the deep emotional impact of a terrible loss by suggesting that moving forward is as simple as "choosing a positive reality." I realize that it is much more complex than that. I am afraid that many find themselves in the most negative reality imaginable from which movement must seem impossible. It is difficult for me to write this because I have not yet experienced that which I imagine to be the worst—the premature loss of a spouse, parent or child to accident or illness. I could never say *I know how you feel,* because I don't, and I would pray that I never would. I can only imagine the throbbing pain of a loss so profound that the effort to simply move forward through the day seems insurmountable. So, all I can say to the parent who has lost a child, or to another who has lost a spouse, is that I am truly sorry for your loss and that I hope you have found peace and acceptance, or are able to, when you are ready.

It is in the metaphysical sense that you need to understand that you have the power to pick your reality. It is not possible for you to pick every probability or reality because, as I just discussed, often you will find yourself in realities, or situations, not of your choosing; but, from that point on, you have the power to choose how to react. If you are faced with two assumptions, one positive and one negative, what benefit is there in choosing the negative? If you are faced with two actions, one positive and one negative, what good is there in choosing the negative? This is the mechanism by which you can change your life. It is essential that you begin a cascade of positive energy by choosing, or *observing*, the positive assumption or positive action.

The most likely outcomes of positive energy are positive consequences. The most likely outcomes of negative energy are negative consequences. You can be positive/optimistic or negative/pessimistic. We all know people of both species; *Homo sapiens positivus* and *Homo sapiens negativus.* Which one are you, *most of the time?*

Every minute of every hour of every day we are faced with an array of assumptions and actions. It may be as simple as turning left or right, or as complex as should I or should I not undergo chemotherapy for treatment of node-negative, advanced tumor stage colon cancer. There may be a significant other that you had a disagreement with and you're wondering, *She loves me, she loves me not.* An estranged child you were supposed to have a dinner with cancels at the last moment; and you might assume that something important came up and he simply couldn't make it, or he maliciously canceled to be hurtful to you.

Remember that this is your life. This is your reality. You may as well make it a good one. You must. Please do not underestimate the awesome power of the mind and positive thought. I am not suggesting that you can control the individual paths of electrons at the quantum level with thought. What I am suggesting is that you can *choose or influence* those more positive electron paths at the quantum level by thinking the positive thought and by performing the positive action, with the results being reflected at the macro level in the world in which we live. It is by harnessing this amalgam of positive energy that we start a chain reaction of positive consequences that becomes a self-fulfilling prophecy of contentment in which anything is possible.

The logic of Euclid

Euclid of Alexandria (300 BC), regarded as the "Father of Geometry," built an entire field of mathematics based upon a set of five axioms by using the power of deductive reasoning or deductive *logic*. This method was exemplified by Sherlock Holmes in the solving of his cases. He would discover clues (truths) and from these clues he would draw logical conclusions (deductions) with which he would build his case and finger the bad guy, *"Elementary, my dear Watson."* In much the same fashion, a medical doctor will evaluate symptoms (location, timing and quality of pain), laboratory and x-ray results (clues) and physical findings on exam (more clues), from which a conclusion (diagnosis) will be made. A simple mathematic representation of deductive logic would be: if $a = b$, and $b = c$, then $a = c$. *Hey, I like this kind of math.*

The five axioms of Euclid represented truths from which other truths could be deduced and from which conclusions could be made. Two of Euclid's axioms that can be simply stated are: two points can be joined by a straight line; and, two lines that are not parallel will eventually intersect if extended long enough. With the application of these basic axioms and three others, Euclid was able to logically construct more truths and solve complicated geometrical problems by applying the rules.

My approach to the first pillar of emotional health has been *Euclidean* all along, as it will be as we move forward into the next two pillars. To begin with, I wanted to establish a possible link between overweight/obesity and emotional health and then I needed to define emotional health, or the lack thereof. I touched upon emotional healing, breaking the cycle of dysfunction, and the culture of *to do good things*. This amounted to my representation of *the problem,* the problem of ill emotional health, of which one of the side effects might be obesity.

Having defined the problem, I needed to establish a set of axioms, or rules, or natural laws with which to solve the problem. This required a basic idea of the following: the structure of an atom, the fundamental forces of the universe, the double-slit lamp experiment, and a discussion of the Copenhagen and many worlds interpretations of the uncertainty principle.

Finally, with the power of deductive reasoning, I have used the axioms to draw conclusions in my attempt to solve the problem.

⚌

The universe is made of atoms.
(*universe = atoms*)

You are part of the universe.
(*you = universe*)

Atoms are made of a nucleus, space and electrons.
(*atoms = electrons*)

Therefore,

You are made of nuclei, space and electrons.
(*you = atoms*)

#

There is uncertainty in regard to the simultaneous
measurement of the momentum and position of an
electron—uncertainty principle.
(*uncertainty = electrons*)

The universe is made of nuclei, space and electrons.
(*universe = electrons*)

Therefore, drawing from all of the above,

The universe is nondeterministic (uncertain).
(*universe = uncertainty*)

#

Your thoughts and your actions are part of the
universe.
(*thoughts = universe*)

Your thoughts and actions are a product of the
fundamental electromagnetic force between atoms.
(*thoughts = atoms*)

Therefore, drawing from all of the above:

(*universe = atoms*) & (*universe = uncertainty*)

Your thoughts and actions are not predetermined.

Or, otherwise stated,

Your thoughts and actions are subject to your own self-will.
(*thoughts = uncertainty = free will*)

✳

I could have said *think positively and be optimistic represents (a), and life will get better represents (c); therefore, a = c.* That is the equivalent of saying, "We-ell… Because," just like Sister Carol. Sorry, Sister. That is not good enough.

I have explained why *a = c* to the best of my ability. I have spent much time on *a = b* and *b = c*, but in order for you to effect a meaningful change I needed to touch you deep inside, to flip an invisible switch, maybe a quantum one, to push you in the direction you need to go, *now*.

First Principle of the Diet Theory of Everything (DTOE)

By thinking and acting positively *you increase the probability* of positive outcomes.

Energy (positive) $= mc^2$

Positive Energy = Happiness

Therefore,

Happiness $= mc^2$

✳

Your thoughts and actions are subject to your own free will (choice).

Thinking and acting positively increases the probability of positive outcomes.

Positive outcomes lead towards happiness.

Therefore,

It is your choice whether or not to travel towards happiness.

⌗

First Step of the DTOE: *Be happy.*

This is logical to a degree that even Spock, of *Star Trek* fame, would find satisfying; although, as a good Vulcan, the highest calling in his life was the complete suppression of all emotion.

> KIRK: You're about to remind me that logic alone dictates your actions?
> SPOCK: I would not remind you of that which you know so well.
>
> *from* Star Trek II: The Wrath of Khan

Like the classical physics of Einstein and the mechanical laws of motion derived by Newton, the first principle and first step of the DTOE mesh with common sense and observation. A positive action will most likely result in a positive reaction. It is like smiling at a stranger as you pass, or saying hello. They will most likely reciprocate. If you are pulling out of a crowded parking lot and stop to let another car pass, it is likely that a following car will stop to let you pass. But these are only elementary examples, my dear reader.

At the current time in our universe, with a deep space temperature of 2.7 degrees Kelvin (–454.81 degrees F), there are only 24 hours in a typical earth day; therefore, you may need to replace an equivocal action, such as watching a rerun of *Seinfeld*, with a positive one, such as a thirty-minute aerobic exercise session *while* watching *Seinfeld*. A positive action could be as simple as never eating another ButterBurger, or as momentous as going back to school or healing a broken relationship.

More significant positive outcomes result from more significant positive actions. This requires effort. The larger the effort, the larger the outcome—Newton's third law—*for every action there is an opposite and equal reaction.*

This is not always easy. It takes constant effort and requires constant awareness, like most things in life that are good. By continually striving to think and act positively you will engender reciprocal responses and reciprocal outcomes. No matter where you start from in your current state of relativity, there is *always* a higher plane of happiness for you to realize—it is all but a matter of choice. It is easy to imagine how this might transform your life, and collectively, how it might change the world.

This first and most important principle works because it is based on the natural laws of our universe—as surely as the speed of light in a vacuum, or the first law of thermodynamics, which we will be addressing in the next section. Your enhanced awareness of our mysteriously beautiful universe and application of the universal truths will give you control of your existence as you guide yourself forward in a positive direction and fulfill your own joyous reality.

DIET

"Energy is mass, mass energy,"—that is all
Ye know on earth, and all ye need to know.
(after "Ode on a Grecian Urn," by John Keats,
the last stanza of which begins:
"Beauty is truth, truth beauty.")

chapter nine

E = mc²

I SINCERELY HOPE THAT YOU found the previous section helpful. Let's assume that we are all emotionally well, or on the way to becoming emotionally well, or at least thinking of taking steps, if even baby steps, in that direction.

This next part I doubt you would find in any other diet book. Much of what you've already read is not common to other diet books, which is why I am compelled to write this one. I don't think it at all extraneous, otherwise I wouldn't write it. I want you to know the *why* and the *how* of lifestyle change and energy balance. It is important to me that you understand why you should do the things I am suggesting; because, if you truly understand, and if you choose to make the proper choices that I will show you, then there is a high probability of success and little excuse for failure.

$$E = mc^2$$

E energy
m mass in kilograms
c the speed of light in a vacuum in meters per second

In 1905 Einstein wrote a paper on the equivalence of matter and energy that grew from his thoughts on the special theory of relativity. $E = mc^2$ has become the most famous equation in all of science and at the very basic level tells us that mass and energy are interchangeable. Mass is simply anything with substance or weight, such as our body mass (weight) as it is applied in the BMI tables. The equation defines energy as mass multiplied by speed (mc^2); and since the speed of light squared is such a large number, 448,900,000,000,000,000 or about 450 million billion miles per hour, there is a great deal of energy in a small amount of matter. This is exemplified by the power of the strong nuclear force contained within the atomic nucleus, which is unleashed in the controlled form of the nuclear energy of a nuclear power plant or the uncontrollable chain reaction of a nuclear detonation.

The joule, as a unit of measure for energy, is a representation of Einstein's equation, because as you can see from the formulaic definition of a joule:

$$1\,J = 1\ kg \times meter^2/second^2$$

it is defined as *mass* (kilograms) times *speed* (meters per second). The potential (stored) energy of a one-kilogram (2.2 lb.) object held 1 meter above the surface of the earth is equal to 9.8 J. Imagine the weight in your hand, about that of three Happy Meals. If this is dropped from

1 meter (39 inches) above the ground, 9.8 joules of potential energy is converted to 9.8 joules of kinetic (motion) energy which is then converted to heat and sound when it hits the earth. If you lift it back up to one meter above the earth, the energy cost will then be 9.8 J.

To put this in perspective, we will compare all energy equivalents to the "nutritional calorie," which is denoted by "Cal" or "Calorie." The nutritional calorie represents 1,000 calories, denoted by a small "c" (gram calorie). The amount of energy required to raise 1 gram of water 1 degree Celsius is the value of the small calorie; whereas, the amount of energy required to raise 1 kilogram of water 1 degree Celsius is 1,000 c, or 1 Cal (nutritional calorie). It is simpler to quantize the nutritional value of food with the larger unit of measure; otherwise, if counting the gram calories in a hard-boiled egg, you would have 75,000 calories instead of the conventional 75 nutritional calories.

In Europe and Australia, the preferred unit of measure of food energy is the kilojoule. Just as the "small" calorie is too small to be practical in the nutritional labeling of the energy content of food, so is the joule too small to be practical for the same purpose.

With this in mind, the value of 1 joule equals 0.00024 Calorie (nutritional). Our one-kilogram weight one meter above the surface of the earth contains 0.0023 Calorie, which is derived from 9.8 joules multiplied by 0.00024 Calorie/joule, of potential energy. One joule is approximately that amount of energy contained in a drop of Guinness. Contrast this with an earlier illustration of the nuclear power unleashed from the 0.0006 kilogram of uranium in Little Boy that resulted in a 12,500-kiloton explosion over the city of Hiroshima. If the 12,500 kilotons is converted to Calories, the equivalent amount is 1.25×10^{10}, or twelve billion, five hundred million Calories.

It may well be that there is a galaxy far, far away, where intelligent beings are able to biologically harness nuclear power by ingesting a BB-sized uranium pellet every twenty years, allowing them to live and function without observing the mundane tasks of urination and defecation. However, as the intelligent beings in this galaxy, our biological systems can only harness the chemical energy from the bonds between atoms, which is much less potent than that within the atomic nucleus.

The primary role for nuclear energy in our universe is that of the thermonuclear fusion of four atoms of hydrogen into one atom of helium that occurs in the stars, including our own, thereby allowing life on this third planet from the sun. A secondary role is, of course, that of a controlled release for the provision of energy for the use of humankind.

Being resigned to the pedestrian power of chemical energy, I thought it would be interesting to illustrate some respective chemical energy values of everyday substances.

Substance	Calories/kg (nutritional)
Gasoline	11,202
TNT	989
Vegetable oil	10,079
Body fat	9,076
Protein	4,000
Carbohydrate	4,000
Nuclear fusion	71,653,768,988
Specific orbital energy of low earth orbit	7,882

From the table you will note that the energy density of the foods we eat is roughly equivalent to gasoline, and the energy of a low earth orbit. Surprisingly, the energy density of TNT is far less. What accounts for the explosive power of TNT is the *rate of energy release.*

Macronutrients

Henceforth, there will be much talk of macronutrients. The general term refers to the organic elements, carbon, hydrogen, oxygen, and nitrogen, which are required for the growth and development of biological systems. I will be using the term in a more global sense when discussing our diet, which is largely composed of the above four elements. There are three macronutrients from which we may derive energy, which are contained in varying degrees in the foods we eat.

The energy value of the three macronutrients,; fat, protein, and carbohydrate, that we consume is derived from the chemical bonds contained within them, which represent sources of potential energy. This stored energy results from the attractive forces between atoms that are formed into molecules, as described by the laws of quantum electrodynamics. Atoms bond together and form molecules by sharing electrons. The chemical bonds represent the attractive force between two or more atoms, which have nuclei that *want to share* their electrons so as to fill the "empty spaces" in their outer orbital shells.

The chemical energy of a chemical bond represents the electromagnetic, fundamental force between electrons and protons; whereas, the nuclear energy of a nucleus represents the strong nuclear, fundamental force that holds together the subatomic particles of the nucleus. The energy required to knock an electron away from an atom is not nearly as strong as the energy required to break up an atomic nucleus.[31]

Each atomic nucleus is surrounded by orbital shells in which the electrons are found or, I should say, where they have the highest probability of being found. There are six possible shells, and only enough room in each shell for a certain number of electrons, all having a unique quantum number of four digits that define a specific space for each electron.

Oxygen, as an example, with an atomic number of eight, has eight protons and eight electrons. Two of the electrons reside in the closest shell, which can only hold two. The remaining six electrons are in the outer shell, which has a capacity for eight. Oxygen, therefore, has two "empty" spaces in its outer shell. As luck would

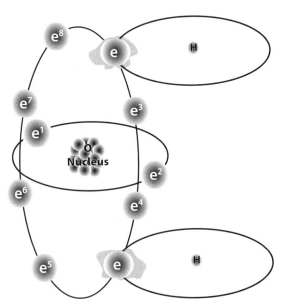

Oxygen sharing its two "empty" spaces with the electrons of two hydrogen atoms to form H_2O (see page 109).

have it, hydrogen, which has an atomic number of one (one proton and one electron), is essentially a *free* electron, with an attached nucleus, and is more than happy to share the empty space of oxygen's outer orbital shell. As there are two empty spaces, oxygen is able to share its outer orbital shell with *two* hydrogen atoms. The attraction of hydrogen's electron to the "empty" space of oxygen's orbital shell is strong enough to overcome the repulsion of the positive charges of the two, now adjacent, nuclei (oxygen and hydrogen). This allows for a fully filled orbital shell, with the maximum of eight electrons—ergo—water. *Building blocks.* Isn't it beautiful in the way it all fits together?

First law of thermodynamics

$dU = \delta Q - \delta W$

dU is an infinitesimal increase in the internal energy of the system

δQ is an infinitesimal amount of heat added to the system

δW is an infinitesimal amount of work done by the system

δ denotes an inexact differential

"The increase in the internal energy of a thermodynamic system is equal to the amount of heat energy added to the system minus the work done by the system on the surroundings."

This is the statement of the conservation of energy, which decrees that energy cannot be created or destroyed. It is a natural law of the universe and is inviolate. Now let me substitute some units of measure more familiar to us.

dU is an infinitesimal increase in body fat mass

δQ is an infinitesimal amount of macronutrient consumed by the system

δW is an infinitesimal amount of exercise done by the system

δ denotes an inexact quantity

"The increase in body fat mass is equal to the amount of energy consumed by you, the system, minus the amount of energy expended by you, again, the system."

To further clarify—the energy expended includes your daily metabolic needs plus the energy expended in watching the 250th rerun of an episode of M*A*S*H, walking to the fridge for another beer, jogging a couple of miles, and everything else it is that you do throughout the day and night. If the energy consumed equals the energy expended, then the infinitesimal increase in body fat mass is zero. *Yeah!* If the energy consumed is less than the energy expended, then there is an infinitesimal *decrease* in the body fat mass. *Double yeah!* If the energy consumed is greater than the energy expended, then there is an infinitesimal *increase* in the body fat mass. *Oh, son of a gun!*

Please forgive my redundancy, but this is so important—if your caloric intake exceeds your caloric output, you gain weight. To explain this to my three-year-old granddaughter eating her sixth sugar cookie, I would say, "Don't eat that, Evie. It'll go straight to your biscuits." It's not rocket science. Okay, maybe it is, but at least it is comprehensible rocket science.

Even if you have a genetic predisposition or a rare bio-logical defect in your DNA, the above holds true. We have already discussed the role of genetics and the obesogenic environment in the overweight and obese. Only a select, unfortunate few are the true mutants: the Mendelian syndromes of which mental retardation is a feature, and the single-gene mutations of which only one or two fami-lies of Middle Eastern descent have been identified. All the rest—*you*—are not mutants and are not predestined to a lifetime of obesity. There are varying degrees of difficulty in maintaining weight in our obesogenic cul-ture; but with the empowerment of knowledge that leads to lifestyle changes, these difficulties will be overcome.

Weight gain is a function of what you eat and what you do. Your daily weight is a reflection of the energy consumed less the energy expended. It is either zero, positive, or negative. When someone tells me that they can't lose weight, that nothing works, do you know what I think? I think that there are three possibilities. Either the individual is not human but, rather, an alien life-form from another universe not subject to the natural laws of this one; or the individual is eating too much and/or not exercising enough; or the individual is not eating or exercising in the right way.

chapter ten

Biological energy systems

I AM AFRAID THAT WE have one more set of building blocks in front of us. Happily, they are built on what we have discussed before and their purpose is to illustrate the chemical energy of the food that we eat. I think it important that you know these building blocks, because when you are fully aware of the energy density (caloric content) of the foods that you eat, and *what that really means,* you will tend to think before you swallow. You will look at a label, do some math in your head and, more often than not, will decide that the energy cost is not worth it. You will be making informed decisions on what you eat, which will have a direct impact on your weight.

♯

Okay. Time for a bit more heavy lifting—please don't get sidetracked by the multiplication and division; there isn't that much, and it's not very long, and it's the last of the tough stuff.

The short answer of what follows over the next five pages is that the food we eat contains chemical energy that our bodies convert to potential energy that is stored in our tissues. When that energy is accessed for metabolism it is converted to a different kind of chemical energy that our body is able to use. That being the case, by now you know my penchant for the longer answer, which I think is so much more interesting, and it is as follows. (If you do opt for the short answer, dear reader, please continue on with the section "Macronutrients" beginning on page 165.)

♯

Everything that we eat can be condensed down to three basic macronutrients: carbohydrates, fats, and proteins. The primary role of carbohydrates and fats is as an energy substrate. Although protein can be metabolized as an energy substrate, as in a fasting state when carbohydrate and fat stores have been depleted, its primary role is that of structure and function. It forms the building blocks of the various organ systems of the body. Only at the end stages of starvation, as in anorexia nervosa, after all of the fat and carbohydrate are gone, after most of the skeletal muscle has been catabolized away, only then is the visceral protein of the liver and heart metabolized for energy, and if too much is taken, death ensues.

The chemical potential energy, residing within the bonds of the macronutrients consumed, is extracted and conserved within the bonds of adenosine triphosphate (ATP) during the body's processes of metabolism. ATP is a large molecule composed of atoms of five elements of differing amounts: carbon, hydrogen, nitrogen, oxygen and phosphorus. This is designated by the chemical formula of $C_{10}H_{16}N_5O_{13}P_3$, which means that ATP has ten carbon atoms, sixteen hydrogen atoms, five Nitrogen atoms, and so on. The chemical energy stored in the molecules of ATP is then used to drive the life-sustaining work of the biological systems. The potential energy within this molecule is responsible for supplying all of the cells' energy for work.

Adenosine triphosphate

The amount of energy released or required for the breaking or forming of the third phosphate bond is 7.3 Calories per mole. This is reflected in the equation:

$$ATP + H_2O \longleftrightarrow ADP + Pi - \Delta G \text{ 7.3 Cal/mol}$$

Hydrolysis of ATP (addition of water). The negative delta sign, Δ, indicates that energy is released (7.3 Cal/mol).

The atomic weight of ATP is derived by adding all the atomic weights of the atoms comprising the ATP molecule $C_{10}H_{16}N_5O_{13}P_3$: carbon has an atomic weight of 12, so there is 120 grams of carbon (10 × 12) in each mole of ATP; hydrogen has an atomic weight of 1, so there is 16 grams of hydrogen in each mole of ATP, and you add up all the rest to reach the total of 507 grams.

The mole is the scientific definition of a unit of substance, which is used to measure a physical quantity of a substance. Each mole contains 6.022×10^{23} "elemental entities," which in this case are *molecules*. This number is known as Avogadro's number, in honor of Amedeo Avogadro, the Italian scientist who first realized that the volume of a gas is proportionate to the number of atoms or molecules within that volume of gas. The Avogadro number is a constant, which means that it is unchanging, and equals the number of atoms in exactly twelve grams of carbon. It can also represent the number of molecules, which is how I have used it above.

The addition of water to ATP is referred to as hydrolysis; therefore, with the hydrolysis of one mole (507 g) of ATP, there is a release of 7.3 Cal of energy for the purpose of biologic work. In the intracellular environment the actual value may approach 10 Cal/mol (507 g). Since the body only stores up to 100 grams of ATP at any one time, the ATP must be continuously resynthesized from the biological burning of the macronutrients, primarily carbohydrate and fat, and, to a lesser extent, protein.

The resynthesis of ATP is made possible by the process of oxidative phosphorylation that is more simply described as biological burning. This process involves the transfer of electrons from large protein molecules to oxygen. It is the energy of these electrons, *which may or may not be in any particular place at any particular time*, moving from one quantum level to another, or from one "shell" to another, that contributes to the resynthesis of ATP. From the previous equation, we know that it requires 7.3 Cal to resynthesize one mole (507 g) of ATP.

The complete breakdown of one mole of glucose $C_6H_{12}O_6$ to the end products of carbon dioxide and water generates 686 Calories of chemical energy. This energy then becomes available to the cell/organism/system/ you. Divide this amount by 7.3, and you would surmise that a total of 93.9 moles of ATP is resynthesized. Alas, we are not one hundred percent efficient and only about 38 percent of the energy is conserved in the phosphate bond formation of ATP, with the remainder being dissipated as heat, which is why exercise makes you warm. The breakdown of one mole of glucose therefore regenerates 36 moles of ATP. This amounts to a total of 263 Calories of free energy gain, which is obtained when multiplying 36 moles by 7.3 Calories per mole.[32]

$$C_6H_{12}O_6 + 6\ O_2 \longrightarrow 6\ CO_2 + 6\ H_2O + 686\ Calories$$

Aerobic respiration of one mole of glucose
to carbon dioxide and water, resulting in release of energy,
exhalation of CO_2 and excretion of water.

This next part is easier.
Now let's be like Euclid and exercise the deductive reasoning muscle between our ears.
Given:

0.00024 Cal = 1 J, and thereby

9.8 J = 0.0023 Cal, and

1 mole of glucose (180 g) yields 263 Cal of free energy gain, and

the potential energy of a 2.2-pound weight 1 meter above the earth = 9.8 J

From the above, one can conclude that the metabolism of one mole of glucose weighing 180 g yields the free energy equivalent of raising, *and lowering* (9.8 J each way), a 2.2-pound weight one meter off the floor about 5,834 times. Not too shabby, unless compared to nuclear fission, in which case it is quite so.

I should clarify—5,834 times in the case of a *weight-less* arm. We need to account for the weight of your arm because that becomes part of the work of lifting. So, assuming that you are physically raising and lowering the weight, and assuming that the weight of your arm is ten pounds, the total weight of 12.2 pounds would come to 1,052 times raising and lowering the 2.2-pound weight.

I know what you're thinking—*no way, 5,834 is a big number, as is 1,052.* So, think of it this way. Using myself as an example because I am exactly 100 kg on a good day and that is the equivalent of one hundred 2.2-pound weights, let us figure out how many calories I expend in jogging. If I have a pace count of 160, meaning that there are 160 foot strikes per minute, and between forward and upward motion I average the equivalent of 0.3 meter (12 inches) above the surface of the earth, then 160 (foot strikes) × 100 (kg body weight) = 1,600 kg weights, lifted per minute 0.3 m above the surface of the earth. This is the equivalent of lifting a 1 kg weight 1 m above the surface of the earth 480 times per minute (1,600 × 0.3). This means that in twelve minutes I have performed the equivalent of lifting a 1 kg weight 1 m above the surface of the earth 5,760 times (12 × 480), which as we know is very close to the cost of 263 Calories. This is almost exactly what my treadmill reads after twelve minutes of jogging at six and a half miles per hour, which for me is a pace count close to 160.

Macronutrients

Carbohydrate

Energy equivalent: 4 Calories per gram.

Simple sugars

Glucose is a molecule containing six carbon atoms which may form a chain or a ring, and has oxygen and hydrogen atoms that are chemically bonded (shares electrons) to each of the carbon atoms. Other sugars are of a similar structure with similar atoms but of differing configurations. Simple sugars are composed of one (monosaccharide) or two (disaccharide) molecules of carbohydrate. Examples of these are listed below.

> **Glucose**—primary carbohydrate energy substrate of mammalian tissues
> **Fructose**—occurs in fruits and honey
> **Galactose**—found in dairy products
> **Lactose**—glucose + galactose
> **Maltose**—glucose + glucose
> **Sucrose**—glucose + fructose; same as table sugar

All glucose is equal, thermodynamically speaking. The amount of energy held within the chemical bonds of a glucose molecule of powdered sugar equals that of a glucose molecule found in a buckwheat pancake. It doesn't matter if you chew a glucose molecule off an organically grown apple or swallow it straight from the test tube of a freshly synthesized sample in the sterile confines of a lab—the energy content is the same.

Technically, an apple doesn't have glucose; rather, it has fructose, which is easily converted to glucose in the liver; and powdered sugar is actually sucrose that is a disaccharide of glucose and fructose. It doesn't really matter which form of carbohydrate is ingested, because the final common pathway for all carbohydrates is the eventual conversion or breakdown into glucose.

Complex sugars

Three to thousands of sugar molecules linked together are called polysaccharides, which include starches. There are two types of starch: amylase, which is a long chain of glucose molecules joined end to end; and amylo-pectin, which is a highly branched polysaccharide, struc-tured like the branches of a tree. Because of the highly branched nature of amylopectin, it is rapidly absorbed (high glycemic index) as there are multiple "ends" to be cleaved off simultaneously; whereas, with amylase, only one glucose can be cleaved off at a time and it is thereby absorbed more slowly (low glycemic index).

Fiber, cellulose, is a structural polysaccharide that is naturally occurring in plants. It does not contribute significantly to the caloric intake because it is not digest-ible by human intestinal enzymes; however, it does slow the absorption of carbohydrates and thus impacts the glycemic index. Foods higher in fiber content have a lower glycemic index due to the slower absorption of glucose.

Glycemic index

High glycemic index—rapidly absorbed, causing immediate surge in insulin.

Low glycemic index—slowly absorbed, causing a delayed, more gradual rise in insulin.

As stated previously, all glucose is equal, thermodynamically speaking, *but some glucose is more equal than others.*
I am referring, of course, to the glycemic index, which
reflects the relative rate of absorption of various carbohydrates and the accompanying surges in insulin. The
two primary factors that determine the glycemic index,
from our above discussion, are the presence of fiber and
the structural form of the carbohydrate itself. It should
be obvious from this that the simple sugars, unadorned
with fiber or burdened by form, would be the most rapidly
absorbed and cause the highest surges in insulin. High
glycemic index foods are not desirable most of the time
for reasons that will be made clear in future sections.

You don't need to know whether a carbohydrate is
highly branched, complex, or simple, although it wouldn't
hurt. You don't even need to know exactly how much
fiber a carbohydrate has, although that is considerably
easier, as it is listed on the container, or can be found
in a calorie/nutrition handbook. In simply understanding the concept of the glycemic index, common sense will
tell you that a glazed donut has a higher glycemic index
than a bowl of bran cereal. As for the rest, familiarizing
yourself with lists of low and high glycemic index foods
will be helpful. Until you find the time to do that, avoid or
restrict the white starches (bread, pasta, potatoes) and
refined sugars (soda and sweets).

Interpreting the glycemic index isn't as simple as
referring to a list, although that is a start. The glycemic index of a particular food is dependent on how it is
prepared, what else is eaten with it, and also the total
amount consumed; for instance, a small amount of a
high glycemic index food would have less impact than
a larger amount of a lower glycemic index food—this is

the concept behind *glycemic load*, which is a calculation of the total glycemic impact of a food consumed. Simply remember that the goal is to limit high glycemic index foods against the backdrop of controlling calories *first*.

Examples of high glycemic index foods

White bread, bagels, doughnuts
Low-fiber cereals: Rice Krispies, Corn Flakes
White potatoes, white rice, corn
Watermelon, cantaloupe, pineapple
Soda, sugar-sweetened sports drinks
Ice cream (low-fat), candy

Examples of low glycemic index foods

Nuts and seeds
Whole grain bread, pita
Bran cereals, oats, buckwheat, barley
Apples, peaches, pears, plums
Sweet potatoes, yams
Milk, yogurt, sugar alcohols

Glycogen

Glycogen is a highly branched, storage polysaccharide of glucose molecules that is found in mammalian tissues. It serves as the major carbohydrate energy source. A well-nourished individual will store about 500 g, most of which is in the muscle, the remainder being in the liver. With physical activity of moderate to high exertion, glycogen is the preferred energy source. After roughly two hours of strenuous activity, the glycogen stores become depleted and the body shifts to fat as the primary energy source; however, without the ingestion of glucose, the exercise intensity will decrease by 50 percent.

The presence of glycogen allows for anaerobic metabolism, which refers to the release of energy from glucose in the absence of oxygen. Anaerobic metabolism occurs with short-term high-intensity exercise such as weight lifting or sprinting—the intensity of the activity exceeds the capacity of the vascular system to supply oxygen, via the blood, to the tissues. This intensity is dependent on a multitude of factors, including hemoglobin level, lung capacity, and the cardiac output, which is a function of heart rate and the amount of blood pumped with each heartbeat.

Glucose molecules are rapidly cleaved off of the glycogen in oxygen-starved muscles, and each glucose molecule is metabolized anaerobically, with the net result being the production of 2 ATP molecules. This is a very inefficient use of glucose, as opposed to the aerobic respiration of glucose that yields 36 molecules of ATP. Lactic acid is the end product of anaerobic metabolism and builds up in the muscles with sustained strenuous activity, ultimately resulting in pain and muscle failure.

The lactic acid that builds up in the muscles is metabolized rapidly as an energy substrate itself, as well as being reconverted back to glucose via a process called gluconeogenesis. The point at which the lactic acid is metabolized as quickly as it is produced is called the lactate threshold—this occurs at different levels of exertion for different people, dependent upon the level of fitness and training. A tenuous equilibrium is sustained until the lactate production exceeds the threshold, resulting in muscle failure. High lactate thresholds are found in endurance athletes, such as iron man competitors, who can maintain their thresholds throughout the course of an eight-hour triathlon.

All carbohydrates go, if not to energy then to fat.

Following absorption from the gastrointestinal tract, glucose is

1. Used as an energy source for cellular metabolism
2. Turned into glycogen in the liver and muscle
3. *Converted to fat* as stored energy—after any existing glycogen deficit is replaced

It is that simple. There is nothing else. Excess glucose does not evaporate from the skin. It is not lost in the stool. It is not excreted into the urine, and if it is—that's bad.

Lipid: fat

Energy equivalent: 9 Calories per gram.

The chemical structure of fat, or lipid, is that of the triacylglycerol (TAG) molecule, also known as triglyceride that has as its basic unit of structure the glycerol molecule. Glycerol is an alcohol made of three carbon atoms, each of which shares a chemical bond with a hydroxyl group (OH). This hydroxyl group, composed of an oxygen atom and a hydrogen atom, is what makes glycerol an alcohol.

The other parts of the TAG are three long chains of carbon and hydrogen atoms, called fatty acids, which attach to each of the hydroxyl groups of the glycerol molecule. During cellular aerobic metabolism (oxygen is required), the fatty acid chains are broken down into carbon dioxide and water, one carbon at a time, yielding a tremendous amount of free energy. The aerobic metabolism of one TAG with three 18-carbon fatty acid chains yields a net of 460 molecules of regenerated ATP.

Some fatty acids are manufactured by the body, but others must be obtained from dietary sources, these being described as the essential fatty acids. When TAGs are digested, the fatty acid chains are separated from the glycerol molecule in the intestine, absorbed, and then reconstituted for transport throughout the body. A significant amount of stored fat, counterintuitively, does not come from ingested fat but, rather, from ingested carbohydrates. Excess carbohydrates are easily and preferentially converted to TAGs—that is the chief available pathway. Excess carbohydrates are not going to be converted into more carbohydrates, because that is what they already are; they are not going to be converted into protein, because protein is obtained from dietary consumption. This leaves only the conversion to fat for all excess carbohydrates not used directly as an energy source.

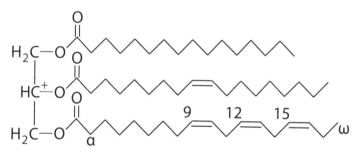

Triacylglycerol. Note the 3-carbon glycerol molecule on the left. The squiggly lines represent the fatty acids that hold most of the energy within their chemical bonds.

Your fat tissue provides as much as 80–90 percent of the energy requirements at rest in a well-nourished individual; however, consider the overfed state in which there are repeated surges of blood glucose and insulin, which encourages fat storage as opposed to fat metabolism. Unfortunately, for an overweight person with a frequent daily consumption of high-calorie, high-carbohydrate drinks, snacks and meals, it is most likely that their fat stores are relatively metabolically inactive, other than for the purpose of increasing the storage of still more fat.

Given an average body fat percentage of 15 percent for males and 25 percent for females, the energy stored in fat ranges from 95,000 to 150,000 Calories in normal-weight adults. Contrast this with the 1,500–2,000 Calories of stored energy in the glycogen reserves, which allows for roughly two hours of exercise. The fat reserves hold enough energy for in excess of 100 consecutive hours of exercise.[33]

Although the glycerol molecule, which is left over after the three fatty acid molecules are cleaved off (*hydrolysis or lipolysis*), can be converted to glucose, the fatty acid molecules do not become substrates for the synthesis of glucose (*gluconeogenesis*). This is important because glucose is the primary fuel for the brain and the red blood cells. If the glycogen stores are depleted and the individual is in a fasting state, muscle protein will be broken down into the substrates for glucose production. Protein can be turned into glucose; fat cannot.

Protein

Energy equivalent: 4 Calories per gram.

Proteins are large molecules made of combinations of smaller molecules called amino acids that are considered to be the "building blocks" of proteins. More than fifty amino acids are found in human tissue. They exist in various three-dimensional configurations, ranging from simple linear arrangements to complex shapes (like pieces of a jigsaw puzzle) that are specific to cellular processes. The amino acids are composed of carbon, oxygen, hydrogen, and nitrogen atoms. Eight of the amino acids cannot be synthesized in the human body and must be ingested; they are known as the "essential amino acids."

Dietary protein is obtained from both plant and animal sources. Unlike carbohydrates and fat, protein is not stored; it is either contributing to tissue structures or is metabolized for energy or stored as fat if consumed in excess. Protein breakdown or catabolism contributes up to 5 percent of the body's total energy requirement; however, with a carbohydrate-restricted diet, protein makes up a larger percentage of the daily caloric needs and becomes a more significant energy source.

Energy considerations of carbohydrate and fat metabolism

Anaerobic metabolism will not carry you far; it is inefficient and miserly when compared to aerobic metabolism. With the addition of oxygen to the system, energy is transferred back to the "spent" ATP, resynthesizing it. The ability of the oxygen atom to accept the electrons of hydrogen atoms makes this possible; the energy transfer occurs, at the subatomic level, all because of the movement of electrons.

In summary, the anaerobic metabolism of one molecule of glucose yields 2 ATP molecules; the aerobic metabolism of one molecule of glucose yields 36 ATP molecules; and the aerobic metabolism of one TAG with three 18-carbon fatty acid chains yields 460 molecules of ATP. The efficiency of fatty acid and glucose metabolism is similar, at 40 percent, with the remainder being dissipated as heat.

Insulin and diabetes

Insulin is a key hormone to be understood. It is an anabolic hormone, which means that it is involved in the process of the "building up" (synthesis) of tissues, as opposed to catabolic, which refers to the process of the "breaking down" of tissues. One of insulin's favorite tissues that it likes to build up is *fat.* The presence of insulin in the bloodstream facilitates the entry of glucose into the body's tissues—muscle, fat, liver—where it is involved in protein and fat synthesis and glycogen replenishment. Insulin is secreted by the pancreas in response to carbohydrate (sugar) ingestion. The carbohydrates are absorbed, raising the blood glucose level, which is then lowered by the action of insulin as the glucose is moved into the tissues.

Another cause of insulin secretion is protein, because as an anabolic hormone insulin not only processes and stores glucose, it also stimulates the synthesis and storage of protein for the purposes of cellular function. This effect of protein ingestion on blood insulin levels is mild in the absence of concomitant glucose (carbohydrate) ingestion; however, if excess protein is ingested with carbohydrates, like at Thanksgiving, then the insulin secretion is markedly accentuated, as much as double that of what it would be with the glucose alone.

Because insulin is an anabolic hormone, it is not involved in catabolism—it *builds up*, not *breaks down*. Because insulin is involved in the synthesis and storage of fat in its efforts to process glucose, it necessarily inhibits the breakdown of fat. In the presence of insulin, fat is made, not metabolized. Conversely, in the absence of insulin, fat is metabolized, not made.

Insulin's priority in its handling of glucose is energy first, glycogen second, and fat third. This means that after any ongoing energy needs have been met, and after the liver glycogen is replenished—typically 50–200 Calories—all remaining glucose, thereafter, is converted to fat for storage. Although most of the body's energy at rest is supplied by fat in the normal case, this can be defeated by an overfed state in which there are persistently elevated levels of insulin, secondary to the ingestion of carbohydrate-rich foods. This allows for a relative suppression of fat metabolism as the primary energy source, in favor of the ingested carbohydrates instead.

The primary defect of type 2 diabetes is a resistance of the tissues to insulin secreted by the pancreas—the pancreas secretes normal amounts of insulin, but the tissues don't respond to it. This is in contrast to type 1 diabetes, in which there is an inability of the pancreas to make enough insulin. The end result is the same—blood sugar is high (hyperglycemia) because the tissues are not responsive to available insulin, as is the case in type 2; or blood sugar is high because there is not enough available insulin, as is the case in type 1. This is why diabetics may require insulin—type 2 because their tissues are resistant and they need more insulin than the pancreas can make, and type 1 because the pancreas doesn't make enough insulin.

Type 2 diabetes is the type associated with the metabolic syndrome and obesity. In the early stages of the disease, the elevated blood sugars and insulin resistance can be treated by dietary modification and medications; however, eventually, if nothing changes, impaired insulin production develops and exogenous insulin (from outside the body) will be required. If change occurs, and by that I mean weight loss—even as little as 10–15 pounds—insulin sensitivity can be restored. The addition of regular exercise will add further improvement of the insulin resistance. Several studies have demonstrated improved insulin sensitivity at the tissue level with exercise, independent of body fat mass.

Recall that most of the body's energy needs at rest are derived from fat metabolism, up to 90 percent, in the normal state. Now consider this in the context of an individual on a high-carbohydrate diet, especially a diet exceeding the daily requirement and rich in high glycemic index carbohydrates. This will lead to frequent and excessive surges in blood insulin levels. As with most things taken to excess, tolerance develops and the tissues become resistant to the insulin and so the pancreas secretes *more* of it.

In this insulin-rich state, with plenty of glucose substrate, the primary source of the body's energy needs shifts from fat to glucose, because fat metabolism is inhibited by insulin. Adding insult to injury, with the still plentiful glucose substrate left over from the dietary influx of white bread, donuts, and Coca-Cola—all the excess is converted to fat. With the increase in body fat, the blood levels of leptin increase proportionately and leptin resistance develops as well, which blunts the urge to *stop eating*, resulting in still more weight gain. The end result is an overweight person who becomes increasingly more overweight and increasingly more insulin and leptin resistant, until one day his pancreas can't make enough insulin, requiring the administration of exogenous insulin. Without proper treatment, the deadly side effects of diabetes will march inexorably forward with endpoints such as hypertension, limb loss, stroke, coronary artery disease and death. It is a vicious and deadly cycle that many are stuck in and many are headed towards.

The encouraging news amongst this scenario of doom and gloom is that it is reversible. And the sooner it is reversed, the better off the individual will be in the long term. As you may have surmised, this involves diet and exercise, but this is not possible unless the proper balance is achieved and lifestyle changes are instituted. You have come far, dear reader, and have worked most diligently—the building blocks are now in place for us to move forward.

Enlightenment requires a comprehension of why a = c, and this is what we have been addressing. We have discussed quantum theory; the equivalence of mass and energy as brought forth by Einstein; the first law of thermodynamics, which states that energy can neither be created nor destroyed; and the energy value of the food that we eat. As creatures of our universe subject to its natural laws, we must become knowledgeable inhabitants and take control of our physical and spiritual selves because no one else can do it for us.

chapter eleven

The relativity diet

THE DIET THEORY OF Everything, more aptly stated as *the thermodynamically sensitive ingestion of macronutrients as a lifestyle change,* is simple. In addition to being simple, it is logical and does not disregard natural law. No expensive supplements are needed. There are no pre-packaged meal plans. You don't check in with anyone, unless you want to; but then you'd have to find an interested party, and that will likely cost money.

Relativity Diet: DTOE = Lifestyle Change ≠ Diet

There are a few broad principles to guide you, with specific directions, cautionary comments, personal anecdotes, and a little science and math sprinkled here and there. For consistency, when examples are required, I will use my own body habitus characteristics, which will range from 220 lb. to 300, depending upon which part of the book we are in.

A Healthy Heart diet, as recommended by the NHLBI, limits the fat intake to less than or equal to 30 percent of the total caloric intake. If this is applied to a 2,400 daily caloric requirement for myself, at 220 lb. (100 kg), the following can be derived:

> **Fat**—a maximum level of *30 percent* of 2,400 Calories is 720 Calories: this equals 80 g of fat.
>
> **Protein**—the recommended amount of 1 g/kg is 100 g total, multiplied by 4, equals 400 Calories. This represents *17 percent* of my daily caloric requirement.
>
> **Carbohydrate**—the remaining Calories are 2,400 minus the 720 Calories of fat, minus the 400 Calories of protein, which equals 1,280 Calories from carbohydrate sources, which amounts to 320 g, or *53 percent* of the daily total.

In the Healthy Heart diet, the lower the fat the better, so the carbohydrate and protein ratios would be higher, *ideally*, according to the NHLBI.

This represents a 53:17:30 ratio of calories obtained from carbohydrates:proteins:fats. The Zone diet as described by Dr. Barry Spears, which is more restrictive of carbohydrates, describes a ratio of 40:30:30. The Atkins diet induction phase limits you to 20 g of carbohydrate per day, which is less than 5 percent of the daily caloric requirement, with the balance being made up of protein and fat, which would be a ratio of something like 4:48:48 of carbohydrates:proteins:fats. The maintenance phase of the Atkins diet is some number less than 120 grams of carbohydrates per day, which in the above example would represent a maximum percentage of the diet from carbohydrate sources of 20 percent as opposed to the 53 percent of the Heart Healthy diet, the 40 percent of the Zone diet, or the 4 percent of the Atkins induction phase.

I've been on all of the aforementioned diets, and they worked for me. I lost a significant amount of weight. Unfortunately, I found them cumbersome and restrictive, and over the course of a few months I regained all the weight that I had lost. Whether your calories are supplied by carbohydrate, fat, or protein is of no matter; the excess is stored as fat, in compliance with the first law of thermodynamics.

What matters are the varying degrees of contributions from the macronutrients, which modulate the metabolic response of your body in different ways, some more desirable than others. This is a key point. There are dietary modifications regarding the timing and manipulation of macronutrients, as well as lifestyle changes, which you can control and that give you the ability to increase your basal metabolic rate significantly, in addition to increasing the mobilization of fat stores. All of these points will be clearly addressed in the upcoming pages.

Classification of diets

The problem with diets is that all diets eventually end. People either meet a goal or they don't. The diet ends; then they resume eating the way they used to—only *more carefully*. Naturally, in most cases this doesn't work and weight is regained. Although many diets are marketed as lifestyle-change diets, they focus mostly on dietary restrictions which rely heavily on meal plans and cookbooks with recipes that may be difficult to follow on a long-term basis. Other diets are quite severe and are intended to be more short-term and aim for a dramatic weight loss inside of two weeks, which invariably involves losing mostly water weight. I am going to attempt a diet classification that is by no means all-inclusive, but many diets will be recognizable to you.

Carbohydrate-restrictive diets

These plans control carbohydrates and fat to varying degrees.

> Atkins
> South Beach
> Zone

Low-calorie diets

These plans have historically focused on caloric intake and counting calories with an emphasis on limiting fat intake, which, by default, means a higher proportion of caloric intake coming from carbohydrate sources. This is the type of diet sanctioned by US governmental agencies. Some of these programs are beginning to modify their approach so as to be consistent with the medical research that is trickling through into the lay media—they are finding themselves in the awkward position of having to address the truth—that there is much more to losing weight than limiting fat. There is nothing wrong with these diets listed below. These diet plans have changed with the times and with the science, but they can be an expensive solution that is a constant reminder that you are on a forced diet, as opposed to a healthy way of eating that is as natural as breathing.

> Weight Watchers
> Jenny Craig

LA Weight Loss
Nutrisystem

Very-low-calorie diets (VLCDs)

These plans are often run by physicians and are severely restrictive and not long-term. There are also many fad diets which periodically seem to make the rounds. A few of these are listed below.

Grapefruit diet
Chicken soup diet
Cabbage soup diet
Mayo Clinic (unofficial) diet: not sanctioned by the Mayo Clinic

Diets difficult to classify

Mediterranean diet—higher in fat content (olive oil), generous with fresh fruits and vegetables and allows moderate pasta and wine intake.

Negative-calorie diet—concentrates on foods that take more energy to digest than the amount of energy consumed—*throw out the cereal, eat the box.*

Three-hour diet—eating every three hours causes a sustained elevation of the basal metabolic rate, which refers to diet-induced thermogenesis (DIT), and is a valid point that will be discussed more fully.

Cookie diet—involves special cookies that control appetite and serve as meal or snack replacements.

One common thread running through most of the above diets is money. They require the use of products: meals, bars, powders, drinks, supplements, etc. What do you think happens when you stop using the products, if they work in the first place? How much do you suppose the monthly cost will run? The weight loss industry is a multibillion-dollar industrial complex that is after your dollar. Beautiful people on the TV screen, with revealing clothes and rippling muscles, will tell you that their product will burn fat effortlessly, without you having to suffer the indignity of changing your eating habits, other than swallowing a few pills daily, for a modest fee of course. Typically, these infomercials promise a thirty-day, money-back guarantee and—*if ordered in the next ten minutes, get two bottles for the price of one.*

Slippage

Have you ever heard of the word *slippage* as applied to this marketing aspect of the retail industry? In financial terms, *slippage* refers to the difference in real and estimated costs. So, if a company makes $3,000 by selling a hundred $30.00 units with a money-back guarantee, there is the estimated potential cost of $3,000 of returns and no net gain, although there still may be some small gain as the cost of shipping and handling is not refundable. Of course, there will not be a 100 percent return of product. The actual cost of refunds to the company for a product that does not work is some number less than 100 percent. That difference is the *slippage*.

How many times have you bought a product on sale for an advertised price that required the submission of a bar code, receipt and rebate form? Do you think everyone does this? I suspect that the slippage in this instance is fairly small, but significant. Not so in the case of mail-order guarantees, which require much more effort, including the passage of time, which typically is thirty days.

Let's say you send away for a few bottles of a sure thing for $29.99 including $12.00 S&H, which you know, from mailing a package just last Christmas, is grossly inflated. Thirty days pass without a loss in weight, now what? You have to look up the address or find the receipt. Then you have to find an appropriately sized box because you were so excited to receive the miracle pills that were going to change your life, like they did for the hard body on TV, that you threw the original box away. Now you have to package everything up and stand in a long line at the post office during business hours and then 15–20 minutes later fork over about five bucks—all this, for thirty pieces of silver. How often do you think this happens, that people actually go through all the bother? *Slippage.*

A recent article published by bankrate.com to the MSN Money Central site[34] summarized the approximate cost to lose thirty pounds, utilizing some popular weight loss programs: Jenny Craig, LA Weight Loss, Nutrisystem, and the Zone diet. The costs ranged from around $400, not including sign-up fees or meals, up to greater than $4,000, which included pre-packaged meals. Most of these listed diets, as well as many others, have modified their plans to include more omega-3 fatty acids and limit exposure to carbohydrates, especially high glycemic index carbohydrates. It's not like it is "special" food. It is just "packaged" food.

You don't need pre-packaged food; it is expensive and not sustainable, unless you can afford it and have a food preparation impediment. And in regard to diet pills, prescription and over-the-counter (OTC), I will address these in detail and whether or not they have demonstrated any efficacy in reputable studies. Realize that weight loss is only a part of your life, a by-product of a healthier life. All it takes is the awareness and implementation of your empowerment, and the resolve and the inspiration to take that first step of *being happy*. It is a gradual process and you are not quite halfway there. You have learned much, but there is still more that I think you need to know about weight loss—this base of knowledge is what I think of as the *relativity diet,* which is kind of like a diet theory of everything (DTOE) in the sense that it encompasses all aspects of the lifestyle modifications that are important.

The diet theory of everything

Most diets rely on restricting calories to varying degrees. Crash or "fad" diets that seem to be popular 7–10 days before a wedding, such as the cabbage soup diet, or all the vegetables and fruit you can eat diet, might limit the caloric intake to around 800 Calories a day, which is a VLCD. Other diets that are meant to be more long-term, such as Weight Watchers, are less restrictive, with daily caloric intakes of 1,200–1,800 Calories, based largely on body size. Carbohydrate-restrictive diets pay less attention to daily caloric intake and focus on limiting the grams of carbohydrates consumed daily.

The DTOE encompasses three components that, when taken together, are much more effective than either alone. This triad includes

1. Counting calories
2. Controlling carbohydrates
3. Modulating metabolism

I am going to emphasize number one, *calories,* because ultimately *calories in equals calories out.* Now, what your body does with those calories is another matter; but, in accordance with the first law of thermodynamics, energy is neither created nor destroyed—*it just is,* from the beginning of time. Therefore, to optimize weight loss we need to control the total calories *in.*

We know that the Calorie (nutritional), as a unit of measure for energy, refers to the amount of energy required to raise the temperature of 1 kilogram of water 1 degree Celsius. This means that if the 273 Calories listed on the nutritional label for a two-ounce Snickers bar is correct, then if the Snickers bar is put in a calorimeter and burned, the result should be 273 Calories. A calorimeter is like a small oven that measures the energy released during the complete combustion of any substance. A calorimeter made by company A in Alberta, Canada, should yield the same result as a calorimeter made by company B in Bogotá, Colombia.

We are all, in effect, calorimeters, in the sense that we burn food as well; but Burt in Bogotá *does not* get the same result as Albert in Alberta. If two different people of the same height and weight and expending the same amount of energy in daily activity consume 10,000 excess Calories over a seven-day period, they will not gain the same amount of weight. This is due to genetic variation and was illustrated by the identical twin experiment, discussed in chapter five, in which twelve pairs of twins received an excess of 84,000 Calories over 100 days and the weight gain varied considerably, especially between unrelated twin pairs, despite everything else being equal.

The uneasy reality is that some people are more prone to weight gain than others and, by default, are less prone to weight loss. A fortunate minority of people are genetically resistant to weight gain and can consume more calories than are recommended for height and weight and still not suffer from overweight and obesity. If you are reading this book, odds are that you are not genetically resistant to weight gain, which means that you are either simply careless in calories consumed versus calories expended, or are genetically predisposed to obesity and not aware of the proper lifestyle changes required for change.

The first, most important task before you is to calculate what your daily caloric need is. Once you know it, then that's it—for the rest of your life. If you are consuming more than the calculated amount and are not genetically resistant to obesity, then you are overweight or obese. If you are a huge Snickers bar fan and eat one 2 oz. bar a day over and above your daily caloric need, you will gain one pound every 13 days because 3,500 excess Calories is roughly equivalent to one pound of fat. After six months, the one extra bar a day amounts to fourteen pounds and, after five years, one hundred and forty pounds. *What? Don't like Snickers? I can't imagine that.* Then substitute a couple of cans of Coke or Mountain Dew or a peanut butter and jelly sandwich or anything else with a caloric value of 273 Calories and you will find the same result. To look at it another way, *if you raise and lower a 2.2-pound weight one meter above the surface of the earth 1,100 times a day,* you will lose the same amount of weight. What would be easier—not eating the Snickers, or lifting a small weight multiple times? What would take the least amount of time?

We will be calculating your daily caloric need. The primary goal is to not exceed this number. In counting and recording the calories that you consume on a daily basis, you are taking responsibility for what you eat; being aware of the caloric content of these foods is crucial. This awareness will serve as a detriment to poor choices. We will be restricting the carbohydrate intake to some extent, in the range of 50–200 grams a day of low glycemic index carbohydrates. This warrants much more discussion and is the topic of a future section. Lastly, we will be increasing your metabolism.

chapter twelve

The science of weight loss

THERE ARE THREE COMPONENTS of our daily energy expenditure: basal metabolic rate, diet-induced thermogenesis, and the energy cost of physical activity. Each of these components can be impacted or modulated in various ways by direct action on our part and therefore deserve further discussion.

Basal metabolic rate (BMR)

There is an energy cost for every breath you take. For every blink of the eye and every beat of your heart—for this and every thought that slips through your mind, there is an energy cost. Just before you awake after a long night's sleep, lying flat under the covers with eyes closed, not too hot and not too cold, that is your basal metabolic state and your body is operating at its basal metabolic rate.

The BMR represents the minimum energy requirements to maintain vital functions in the resting state. It
is most commonly calculated based on body surface area
and is therefore expressed in units of energy (Calories),
surface area (meter^2), and time (hour). The BMR is measured under fairly strict and standard conditions—after
a twelve-hour fast and thirty minutes of rest. A more
relaxed measurement of the BMR is the resting daily
energy expenditure (RDEE), or resting metabolic rate
(RMR), which requires only four hours of fasting and
would be the equivalent of assuming the horizontal
position on your sofa and watching the History Channel.
The RDEE is within five percent of the BMR. Because the
RDEE is easier to calculate, it is used interchangeably
with the BMR.

The BMR can be measured scientifically, in the lab, by
measuring the oxygen consumption over a set amount
of time. This is one of the ways to get a more specific
individualized measurement of the BMR. Another way
to scientifically measure the metabolic rate involves
the ingestion of "doubly labeled water." Participants
in the studies utilizing this technique don't know that
it is special water since it looks and tastes the same.
What makes this water different is a specific quantum
mechanical aspect. It has "heavy" hydrogen (deute-
rium), with an extra neutron in its nucleus, and "heavy"
oxygen-18, with two extra neutrons in its nucleus. The
extra neutrons act as "tags" and can be tracked in the
expired carbon dioxide and water, to thereby arrive at
estimates of energy expenditure.

For most people, who don't have access to a physiology lab, or hydrogen and oxygen with extra neutrons,
the BMR and RMR are estimated from tables of height

and weight, which estimate an individual's total body surface area. Studies utilizing the sophisticated methods discussed above have demonstrated that the BMR or RMR is fairly consistent, relative to the body surface area, when age and gender are accounted for. The lean body mass, fat-free mass (FFM), also correlates well with the BMR, but this is more difficult for off-the-shelf use, as it requires an accurate measurement of the body fat percentage, which can be measured a number of ways, one of the more simple being skin fold thickness. Once the body fat percentage is known, the fat mass can be calculated, which is then subtracted from the total body weight—using myself as an example: my FFM would be 15 percent (body fat) multiplied by 220 lb., which yields 26.4 lb.; therefore, my FFM is 220 less 26.4, or 193.6 lb.[35]

Now that we have an understanding of the BMR, let us discuss how we can change it to our benefit. Our goal, with weight loss in mind, is to effect a chronic elevation of the BMR so that more calories are expended, resulting in a net energy deficit at the end of the day, week, or month, which translates into weight loss. There are two ways in which we can directly impact our own BMR. Both ways involve exercise, each having an immediate energy cost; however, the long-term effect is that of a sustained increase in the BMR.

Increase in FFM

Muscle tissue has a higher BMR than fat tissue; therefore, we can increase our metabolic rate by increasing our muscle mass—lean body mass—FFM. This is accomplished with resistance training and will be fully addressed in the third pillar. As little as one to two hours a week will significantly increase the FFM. A regular program of resistance training will increase the BMR by 5–10 percent, and more, if you really like to lift weights.

The gradual slowing of the BMR, associated with aging, is one of the factors accounting for the insidious increase in weight. The slowing in the BMR is thought to be related to the loss of lean body mass. Implementation of a resistance training program can interrupt and reverse this undesirable process.[36]

Aerobic activity

Resistance training is an anaerobic activity. The muscular contractions occur without the benefit of oxygen because the contractions are too intense and rapid for the lungs and heart to keep up with the transfer of oxygen to the muscular tissues involved. The equivalent of this is sprinting—Olympic sprinters have a very heavy musculature that reflects their anaerobic training, which concentrates on short bursts of intense physical exertion, occurring over a course of seconds to minutes. The marathon runner has a completely different body habitus, which reflects their reliance on aerobic metabolism, occurring over a course of hours.

Aerobic training can increase the BMR by 10 percent, independent of FFM. This means that the 10 percent increase achieved with aerobic training *is over and above* the 5–10 percent that can be achieved with resistance training. The combination of aerobic and anaerobic training represents the potential of a nearly 20 percent chronic elevation of the BMR, which amounts to 300–400 Calories a day in the average adult.

Before your lip curls in disgust because—*of course, that's exercise*—realize that this is not a huge investment of time and effort. It is quite manageable and is one of the positive actions you must make in choosing the reality that you wish to fulfill.

Do obese people have a lower BMR?

Before we leave the topic of the BMR, I would like to dispel a perception that some people hold, and that is—*I am overweight because I have a lower BMR than those who are not obese.* This commonly held perception hearkens back to our discussion on the *set point theory*, the summation being that, although there is no biological set point, there may be an environmental or emotional one.

The question posed is obviously not true; otherwise, I wouldn't be making such a point of it. Assuming that you are not hypothyroid, which is a relatively safe assumption, your BMR should be in line with the available charts and tables.

A study published in the journal *Obesity*, January 2008, addressed the question of whether or not a low RMR was a factor in weight gain and obesity.[37] A total of twenty women, ten obese and ten non-obese, participated in the fourteen-day study. The results demonstrated that the RMR was similar in both groups and that the obese group was more sedentary and expended less energy than the non-obese group. The difference in daily energy expenditure amounted to 300 Calories each day. During the course of the study, the subjects didn't change their normal patterns of activity or diet. Furthermore, the daily energy intake was similar between the two groups, the primary difference being the daily energy expenditure. The increased activity of the non-obese included more time spent standing, as opposed to sitting, as well as roughly 50 percent more time in light and moderate

activity, which included housework and other activities of daily living. The obese subjects were not heavier
because they had lower basal metabolic rates; they were
heavier because they were less active.

DIT

So I can raise my BMR by nearly 20 percent by making a
healthy and positive change in my life—*but I want more.*
That would be DIT. Consider it a bonus. DIT reflects the
metabolic cost of digestion of the various macronutrients.
After a meal, the basal metabolic rate increases as the
body "works" to process the macronutrients, whether it
be for metabolic needs or energy storage. This increase
can be measured as a fraction of the calories ingested,
which varies with each macronutrient. The DIT values are 0–3 percent for fat, 5–10 percent for carbohydrate, 20–30 percent for protein and 10–30 percent for
alcohol.[38,39]

Of the three macronutrients, apart from alcohol, the
largest DIT effect is seen with protein at 20–30 percent;
therefore, if you increase your protein intake as a percentage of your daily caloric requirement, then you will
accentuate the caloric cost of DIT. The increase in calories of protein will come at the expense of carbohydrates
and fat, which is generally a good thing.

The generous effect that protein has on DIT is higher
than in actuality because rarely do we eat solely protein.
Other studies have demonstrated a more modest effect
of DIT in a typical mixed diet (protein, carbohydrate and
fat) of around 10 percent over twenty-four hours; however, it is accentuated with a larger protein fraction.[40]

A simple way to increase your protein intake would
be by eating pickled turkey gizzards instead of rice

cakes as an afternoon snack. I love turkey gizzards, pickled pork hocks, and beef jerky too, so this is easy for me. A general rule I have for snacks is that I try to eat something that has at least as much protein as net carbohydrates. A convenience that I avail myself of often is peeling the wrapper off of a high-protein, low-carbohydrate snack or meal bar that costs from a dollar to a dollar fifty. A typical snack bar of 140 Calories might have 15 g of carbohydrates, with 3 g of fiber, for a net carbohydrate load of 12 g, and 10 g of protein. If I don't have any pickled pork hocks nearby, I'll reach for my pack of whole grain, low-carbohydrate tortillas. Each has 100 Calories, 13 g of carbohydrates with 7 g of fiber and 8 g of protein. One tablespoon of peanut butter and a dollop of sugar-free blackberry jam later, I'm softly chewing my way to satiety. You can find foods that you like that are higher in protein, and this is the way to maximize DIT; the concomitant decrease in carbohydrates can only help.

The DIT effect lasts several hours after eating, but peaks at around one to three hours; therefore, if you eat something every three hours, especially a higher-protein something, then you will have a sustained DIT effect throughout the entire day. Wow! *You mean I have to eat every three hours? Like I said to my drill sergeant in basic training—"Thank you, Drill Sergeant—may I have another?"* You do yourself no favors by fasting. Skipping breakfast is bad, bad, bad. You have already been fasting during the night, six to eight hours at least, depending on a nighttime snack, and by adding another six you have effectively been fasting for more than half of the day. Fasting suppresses the BMR and is counterproductive to our chosen reality. Do not fast!

Believe it or not, there is still more. Exercise aug-
ments DIT. It is approximately doubled. Therefore, if you
exercise, like going for a swim, one hour after eating—
remember that when you were little?—then the metabolic
cost of that exercise is increased due to DIT.[41]

The cost of physical activity

Daily physical activity is the most significant component
of daily energy expenditure, assuming, of course, that
there *is* physical activity. The effects of aerobic exercise and resistance training have been briefly discussed
above and will be fully elucidated in the third pillar:
energy expenditure.

That's it. You have the ability to gradually increase
your BMR over the next six to eight weeks such that it
could be 30 percent or more than it is right now. After
knowing all this, how can there possibly be an epidemic
of obesity in the world today? *Absence of knowledge.*
Knowledge equals empowerment, which equals action.
If I were to stop right here, this would be enough for
most people to gradually return to an appropriate body
weight. But, of course I won't stop, because it is not in my
nature. I need for you to know more. Now I am going to
help you along on the way to your own chosen reality. It
is time to branch off of your current universe to enter
a parallel one filled with positive energy, happiness and
weight loss.

Daily caloric requirement calculation

What we need to do is to figure out what your daily
caloric requirement is, not in your current overweight
or obese state but, rather, at your healthy body weight
state. Therefore, it does not matter how much you weigh

now; it matters *how much you want to weigh in the future*. You need to know what an appropriate Body Mass Index is for you, and this depends on your body frame size. Please refer back to the BMI tables and frame-size estimation methods in chapters three and four. Place bookmarks so they will be easier to find.

Determining appropriate BMI

From the table in chapter three, you will note that the "normal" weight BMI is from 18.5 to 24.9. For a medium or large frame, or a well-muscled small frame, 24.9 will be too low. What we are talking about is a range of values. I would suggest aiming towards the higher end of the range, since any number within that range will be an improvement from where you will be starting. Once you achieve the targeted BMI, which you will, then you can re-evaluate where you are.

If you have a medium to large frame, pick a number between 25 and 30: 30 if you have a large frame and will end up looking like Arnold Schwarzenegger in the movie *Conan the Barbarian;* 25 if you have a medium frame and will end up looking like John Travolta in the movie *Saturday Night Fever;* or pick any number in between, based on the two extremes. If you have a small frame, pick a normal BMI number between 18 and 25.

Determining daily caloric need

After you know what you should weigh, it is a relatively simple matter to calculate your RMR and your daily caloric needs. If you perform an internet search on "formula for caloric expenditure" you will find multiple sites with various formulas and calculators that will calculate your daily caloric requirement. Most of these are based on the body surface algorithms referenced earlier. You will find that all of the calculators will yield a result that will be close to the simple formula of your weight (in pounds) multiplied by eleven. This is an estimation of the daily caloric need for a sedentary adult.

Body Wt. (lb.) ____ × 11 = ____ = Daily caloric need
for *Homo-sapiens sedentarius*

This formula accounts for a sedentary lifestyle by multiplying the BMR by a factor of about 1.2 to get a number slightly higher than the BMR, to account for at least getting out of bed in the morning. Some other formulas use a higher factor, most commonly 1.3.

Take myself, as an example. I am 75 inches tall and, according to the anthropometric tables, have a medium frame. I plan on being fairly muscular, although not to the Schwarzenegger standard, so I'll pick a BMI of 28, which equals a weight of 216 to 224 lb. I'll split the difference and declare my targeted weight to be 220 lb., which is exactly 100 kg—*how convenient.*

My daily caloric requirement equals 220 × 11 = 2,420 Cal.

What is your daily caloric need?

Calculate it now. Write it down. You need to know this.

Real-world applications of the cost of a Calorie

One Calorie is the energy required to raise 1 kg of water one degree Celsius. *Hmmm, that tells us a lot—how about some real-world applications of the Calorie?*

We are physiologically trapped—trapped in the latter portion of the Pleistocene epoch, sixty-five million years after *T. rex* breathed his last. This time, 200,000 years ago, was that of the mammoths, mastodons and saber-toothed tigers. It was a time when *Homo sapiens sapiens* diverged from *Homo erectus*, as a path diverged in the wood.

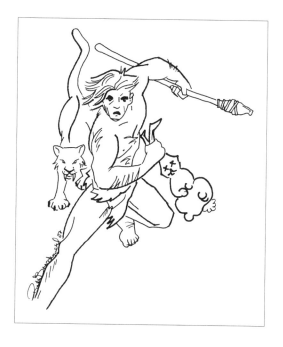

The previous two million years of evolution had been predicated upon the scarcity of food and the metabolic conservation of energy, culminating in the wonderfully efficient fat cell. The fat stores of *H. sapiens sapiens,* replenished in times of plenty, could allow weeks of survival on nothing much more than water. The diet, when there was one, consisted of meat, vegetables, meat, berries, meat, occasional fruit, and more meat. Our ancient ancestor had to run faster than a tight end in the NFL just to catch his next meal. He needed the sinewy strength of a triathlete to scale a rock face and escape the charge of a mastodon or to reach the safety of his cave. This was a time when men were real men—lean, mean and hairy, and women were, well, just a gentle club-bonk away.

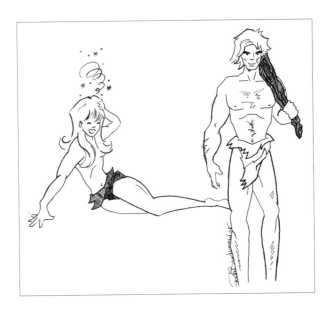

In our current Holocene epoch, the woolly mammoth and saber-toothed tigers are no more. In the last 10,000 years we have shifted from a hunter-gatherer society to an agricultural society. In the past sixty years, white bread, refined sugars, corn syrup, and highly branched complex carbohydrates have become cheap and easy. Instead of chasing down our next meal, we simply stop by the grocery store or the nearest drive-through. We don't need to leave our cars. Motorized scooters zip us up and down the aisles if we're too obese to walk. Remote controls relieve us of the burden of getting up from the couch to change the channel on our TV set. Online ordering of groceries obviates the need of even making the effort to rise from a chair other than to transfer the groceries from the countertop to their respective positions in the kitchen.

Barring a non-motorized crossing of the Sahara desert, a transatlantic paddle in a kayak, or mushing your way across Antarctica on a dogsled, there is little need for the storage capabilities of fat. Obesity did not exist in *H. erectus* or our earlier *H. sapiens sapiens* relatives. It does not exist in the wild today, unless it is meant to— such as the hibernating grizzly bear who will gain several hundred pounds of fat prior to the winter, or the ruby-throated hummingbird that weighs an eighth of an ounce and will add enough fat for the 500-mile crossing of the Gulf of Mexico in its migratory journey south.

We have comfortably conquered Darwin's theory of natural selection and "survival of the fittest." We will not evolve significantly because of the societal enabling and support of obesity in the form of pharmacological treatments of diabetes, cardiovascular heart disease, and hypertension. Even if we did not do this and allowed all of those afflicted to succumb to obesity-related illnesses, it would take a million years or more for our small bowel mucosa to evolve to the point where it would absorb some smaller fraction of the current absorptive quotient, thereby decreasing the efficiency of our intestinal tract, so that we could eat more and not get fatter.

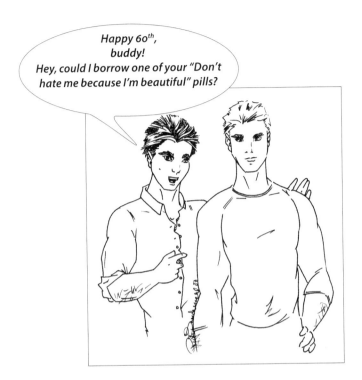

What is more likely is that, as is already happening, there will be pharmacological advancements that will subvert the natural law and allow us to live longer, thinner, prettier, happier, more amorous lives. BUT, until that day comes, that quixotic time when you step out of your modular dwelling unit in the sky to mingle with all the other beautiful people, most of whom have spent half the night making pharmacologically assisted love, we must face one unpleasant fact.

1 pound of fat = 3,500 excess Calories

Some of you may have been *doing the math* and have realized that if fat contains 9 Calories per gram and 1 lb. has 454 g, then doesn't 9 × 454 = 4,086 Cal?

No, because a pound of fat is not all fat; it includes 10 percent water. Additionally, not all fat is absorbed and 5 percent is lost in the feces; therefore, this fifteen percent difference means that roughly 3,500 Cal actually counts towards loss or gain.

Note: In scientific circles the *small calorie* or gram calorie is designated as *cal* (with a small c) and the large Calorie or kilogram calorie is designated as kilocalorie (kcal); whereas, in nutritional applications the large calorie is customarily designated as Cal (with a capital C) and represents 1 kcal, or 1,000 small calories. The gram calorie represents the amount of energy required to raise 1 gram of water by 1 degree Celsius.

Ah, most excellent, sounds like a lot of calories for one pound of fat. *Surely, I don't consume thousands of extra calories a day.* Uh-oh, wait a second, look at how small a Calorie really is as a measurement of energy and power. Another definition of energy is the ability to do work, with the measurement of energy being a Calorie, joule, or foot-pound. Work is defined as force times distance, so you might say that work is involved every time you move yourself from here to there, *or in lifting a 1 kg weight 1 m above the surface of the earth.* Power is defined as the rate of doing work and is measured in watts, horsepower, or Cal/sec, or, in other words, how fast you can move yourself from here to there, or raise and lower that 1 kg weight. Now, let's put these thousands of calories into perspective.

Last fall I picked up a three-horsepower weed whacker at Sam's Club to use on my maintenance-free yard. *Hmmm, a paradox*—why do I need a weed whacker for a maintenance-free yard, you might ask? While it is true that I don't have a lawn mower, I am sorry to say that I own a plethora of hoes, sprinklers, rakes, garden utensils, axes, and a Husqvarna chain saw that triggers gory images of raggedy flesh every time I pull the starter cord. When we built our home five years ago, I laid down the law, as lord of the manor: "There shall be no grass"— *and it was so.* I insisted that our home meld seamlessly with the forest in which it was raised. "I want it to be completely natural," I told Sue, overriding her inclination for a small manicured lawn—*and it came to pass.*

The only problem with my declaration declared itself with the first of the multiple, heavy spring rains that are endemic to Northeastern Wisconsin. All the wood-chip mulch that was spread around the house, in a three-inch layer, to cover the denuded topsoil and fill was promptly washed down the hill upon which our house was built. Along with the natural cedar chips, which were not inexpensive, went a goodly portion of our nutrient-poor soil, causing Sue to say "I told you so." I stood stoically before her, in the mud—*and I saw that it was not good.* Thirty thousand dollars of landscaping later, we were able to keep our bark on top of the hill, but this required multiple, very unnatural, terraced planting beds, interspersed with huge limestone slabs—"Hardscape," said our landscaper. Sue became quite the gardener and I became quite the gardener's helper, especially since I was so much stronger than said gardener.

"Honey, would you please carry these ten bags of peat moss down that hill and up to the other side?"

"Yes, dear."

"Sweetie, you're so big and strong." She'd smiled prettily. "I would really love a raised, fieldstone planting bed at the bottom of the side garden."

"Yes, dear."

"We sure could have fun with an outdoor shower," she suggested on a sultry summer evening in a raspy Kathleen Turner voice, "wink, wink, nod, nod, know whad ah mean, know whad ah mean."

"Yes, dear."

The requests dropped from her lips, as raindrops from the sky. And so on one particular ninety-degree August day I found myself clinging to the side of the cliff, on which our house stood, sunburned, sweaty, and caked in the milkweed scum vomiting forth from the twirling cable of my 3 hp weed whacker as I cleared a swath for some wildflowers she wanted. From where I was perched, I could see Sue up the hill, gardening. She looked pretty in her well-worn cowboy hat as she kneeled in the shade of the side garden while tending to some recently trans-planted black-eyed Susans. Intermittently, she paused to sip from a tall glass of iced tea, the sides foggy and wet from the condensation of hot, humid air on ice-cold glass. Meanwhile, for the past thirty minutes I had been wielding my two-stroke, three-horsepower weed whacker much as King Leonidas must have wielded his broadsword at Thermopylae. How many Calories do you suppose that represents for the weed whacker, whirling away? Let's do the math.

$$\frac{1 \text{ cal/sec}}{0.0056 \text{ hp}} \times \frac{1 \text{ Cal}}{1,000 \text{ cal}} \times 3 \text{ hp} \times 1,800 \text{ sec} = 964 \text{ Cal}$$

The result of 964 Cal is about a third of a pound of fat, had the weed whacker been running on adipose tissue rather than the unleaded 87 octane, plus a little thing of oil I'm supposed to put in every two gallons—*or is it five?*

Looking at it another way, that's one me-sized piece of cheesecake.

The more pertinent question is: How many Calories did I burn during that half hour of absolute torture in the hot sun, with a heart rate of about eighty-five beats a minute? I'd guess a couple of hundred, tops, over and above my basic caloric expenditure—the equivalent of a frosty mug of Guinness stout that I'd toss back in a jiffy, which brings us to the second principle of the Diet Theory of Everything (DTOE).

Second Principle of the Diet Theory of Everything

It is much easier to consume 3,500 Calories than it is to lose it.

I have this friend that we'll call Cal, which is not short for Calorie but, rather, for *calf* because Cal *loves* whole milk. He refuses to drink skim, much less 2 percent, and, God forbid, water. No, Cal's water intake is limited to whatever he gets from Mountain Dew and orange juice. Cal's minimum intake of whole milk and Mountain Dew is one quart and ten cans, respectively, daily. You might have guessed by now that Cal is morbidly obese, and diabetic as well but doesn't know it yet because he hasn't seen a doctor in over ten years. Surprise, surprise, Cal's two boys also drink whole milk and Mountain Dew, and they also are overweight and on a trajectory to morbid obesity.

Cal's idea of dinner is a Meat Lover's pizza, burgers, or any other red meat; his favorite vegetable is the potato, preferably in the form of French fries or chips. His only other vegetable intake is limited to the stray chunk of cellulose that he accidentally swallows with large spoonfuls of chunky beef stew. I don't think Cal goes more than three hours without eating something; unfortunately, the mildly induced DIT effect of fat and carbohydrate does not significantly negate the caloric load. To add insult to injury, the only exercise he gets is the mild activity associated with his job.

Cal is an important person in my life, and it saddens me to see him so unhealthy. I have talked to him obliquely about my feelings, but it is like water off a whale's back because Cal suffers from a distorted body image. He views his obesity as more of an inconvenience rather than the significant threat to his health that it is. In a phone conversation just this evening, as I was writing this, he called to say that he had to see his doctor about an obesity-related health issue. Cal told me that he admitted to the doctor that he knew he had a weight problem, which he (Cal) described as being "pleasantly plump." Cal told me that the doctor said that no, he wasn't "pleasantly plump" but that he was really fat and downright obese and not just obese, but extremely, morbidly obese. I guess the doctor was being emphatic in an attempt to shock Cal back to reality.

The reason I mention Cal is for an illustration of the impact of one small change. Okay, maybe not that small for Cal, but still not at all draconian, and that would be the swapping out of whole milk and Mountain Dew for skim milk and diet Mountain Dew or bottled water.

Values

1 quart whole milk =	600 Cal	32 g fat
1 quart skim milk =	360 Cal	1 g fat
Difference =	240 Cal	31 g fat

$$10 \text{ cans Mountain Dew} = 1,700 \text{ Cal}$$
$$10 \text{ cans diet Mountain Dew} = \qquad 0 \text{ Cal}$$
$$\text{Difference} = 1,700 \text{ Cal}$$

Calculations

Extra Calories per year from whole milk
= 240 × 365 = 87,600 Cal

Extra Calories per year from Mountain Dew
= 1,700 × 365 = 620,500 Cal

Total caloric "cost" of whole milk and MD per year
= 708,100 Cal

Given: 3,500 Calories per one lb. of fat

Potential body fat loss
= 708,100 ÷ 3,500 = 202 lb.

This would drop Cal from morbidly obese to simply overweight—by changing only these two things and nothing
else. I don't think this is too much of a sacrifice, but Cal
doesn't see it that way. He tells me that he doesn't care
for the taste of diet soda, and he said that he read somewhere that diet soda causes Alzheimer's.

This represents a huge daily change in Cal's energy balance—a swing of 2,000 Calories. When I say energy
balance, I mean to say the energy consumed less the
energy expended in the activities of daily living and exercise—this pertains to the first law of thermodynamics
that I so belabored earlier. For most people, weight gain
and weight loss are much more gradual. The effect of the
energy balance is cumulative, and a small mismatch one

way or the other will lead to significant changes over the course of time.

As we age and our BMR slows with the gradual decrease of lean body mass, assuming we are not participating in a resistance training program, if nothing else changes, we gradually gain weight. A loss of one pound of lean body mass represents a decrease in energy expenditure of about 10 Cal a day, which equals one pound per year, *per pound lost of lean muscle tissue.* How much does this add up to over the course of ten, twenty, thirty years?

Consider how significant a 100-Calorie swing in the energy balance would be over time, whether the imbalance is due to dietary change or exercise—skipping that iced latte on the way to work or taking a thirty-minute walk over the lunch hour. A one-hundred-Calorie net deficit per day amounts to about a pound a month, twelve pounds a year and sixty pounds in five years. Obviously, a hundred-Calorie *surplus* per day goes in the other direction as well.

Second Step of the Diet Theory of Everything:
Calculate your daily caloric intake.

$$\text{body weight in lb} \times \frac{11\ \text{Cal}}{\text{lb} \times \text{day}} = \text{Cal/day}$$

$$\text{You (\_\_\_ lb} \times 11) = \underline{\quad} \text{Cal/day}$$

Write it down if you didn't do so earlier. This is so important that I am writing it twice.

This is the *total* caloric requirement/day. The 11 Calories per pound per day represents the RDEE, plus the caloric cost of a sedentary lifestyle which might amount to 500–1,000 Calories over and above the RDEE.

Remember our discussion of various ratios? Well, *don't worry about it.* This is supposed to be easy. The only thing you need to track is the total caloric intake; the rest will follow naturally. By following the general guidelines of low carbohydrate and good fat, you will be "forced" to eat plenty of protein, which, as you recall, carries the highest caloric cost in regards to the DIT effect.

The minimum daily protein requirement, for maintenance of lean body mass, is 0.8 g per kg body weight. At my previous weight of 136 kg this amounted to 109 g of protein per day, which equals about 16 oz. of protein (7 g per oz.). This can be obtained by eating five to eight pieces of chicken, depending on the size of the chicken, (one whole breast, 2 thighs, 2 drumsticks and a couple of wings), which pert near equals a whole chicken *per day.* At my healthy weight of 100 kg I can get by on less than a chicken a day—let's say five chickens a week, not counting the wings, or say seven chickens a week if I just eat the extremities, since I like dark meat better anyway.

Third Principle of the Diet Theory of Everything

The natural tendency is to underestimate the daily caloric consumption of macronutrients.

Third Step of the Diet Theory of Everything:
Record your daily caloric intake, RELIGIOUSLY!

Many dieters drop the ball right here. They make *mental notes* of what they ate, to recall later, if they recall at all—too often, it is a *partial recall.* Total recall only comes from a total recording of *everything.* This is vital and serves three purposes.

1. It forces awareness on you of the caloric cost of various foods, and after 4–6 weeks you will know how many Calories a specific macronutrient holds because you have looked it up so many times before. Additionally, people have food preferences and tend to eat the same things from day to day, so this chore becomes easier to do as time goes on.

2. The awareness of the caloric content of, for instance, a Krispy Kreme Chocolate Brownie Deluxe (300 Cal) will be a detriment to its digestion. You will think hard about whether or not it is worth it to let something past your lips that you know is antithetical to your chosen lifestyle.

3. You will have what you need to effect a meaningful lifestyle change—an accurate count of your calories, not subject to the uncertainty of your brain's electrons on loan from the well of the universe.

There are multiple ways in which to accomplish this. The important thing is to keep a written or other hard record. My wife used an Excel spreadsheet that she kept minimized on the kitchen computer—she recorded her calories in that fashion. I would keep track of my calories throughout the day on an index card, then enter that into the Excel spreadsheet, that Sue made for me, at the end of the day. With PDAs, digital pen recorders, smart cell phones, it has never been easier to keep a record of your daily caloric intake.

Fourth Step of the Diet Theory of Everything: Monitor yourself, *but not too frequently!*

Weighing yourself is more important for some than for others. Sue didn't weigh herself, as you know; she just bought smaller clothes every two months and donated her old ones, *which were actually new,* to the thrift stores. Since she has been at her target weight, Sue has resumed weighing herself monthly. I weigh myself once a week, on Wednesday morning, just after I take care of the daily business. You should weigh yourself *no more than once a week*, and once a month may be even better.

I would also encourage taping, as this may demonstrate results not revealed by loss of body mass. Every month I measured my neck, chest, waist and hips; I found the gradual improvement to be both rewarding and motivating. Given the active metabolism of central or visceral fat, the waist size is one of the first measurements to demonstrate improvement. If you are exercising concurrently with your caloric restriction, as you should be, you can anticipate an increase in lean body mass. Given that lean body mass (muscle) is heavier than fat— *remember that it also has a higher metabolic rate*—your weight loss may not be as dramatic as your decreased measurements would suggest.

Remember this:

The longer you diet, the more fat is lost. In the first week of a negative caloric balance, about 70 percent of the weight loss represents water, which may account for an early impressive result, especially if you start on a day during which you are well hydrated and with full glycogen stores. In weeks two and three of calorie deficit, the percentage of weight loss representing fat accelerates from

25–70 percent, and by the fourth week body fat represents up to 85 percent of the weight loss.[14]

Counting calories

Here are a few other important considerations in regard to counting calories that I will now address.

Scale

In order to accurately count your calories, you will need a digital scale for the kitchen counter at home. These are inexpensive and convenient. All you have to do is put your plate or measuring cup on the scale and turn it on—it will zero and then record only the weight of the food placed on the plate or in the cup. You would be surprised at how little one two-ounce serving of dry pasta is.

Calorie fat and carbohydrate counter

I have a small book that fits into a pocket and cost less than 10 dollars. It lists calories for common and uncommon foods, as well as restaurant chains. There are also digital databases and logs for PDAs (www.calorieking.com/palm/) that are available.

The easiest thing to do is to have some idea or plan of what you are going to eat during the day. I will take meal replacement and snack bars with me if I am going to be out of the house for several hours, in the event that I do not find a suitable alternative.

Portion size

This is where the scale comes in. It is crucial that you weigh your portions of food that are not specifically labeled. After a time you will come to recognize the approximate size of a 4 oz. equivalent of a fish fillet or other low-fat protein source. You will learn that a 2 oz. serving of pasta (dry) is about half a cup. It is easy to let the portion size get away from you at first, but, as your body changes, so will your conceptualization of a properly proportioned meal.

It is amazing what food vendors consider as one portion. You know that medium-sized bag of Ranch flavored Doritos that you get to the bottom of before the first quarter of a football game—how many calories do you suppose that is? Try 1,500 Calories on, try it right on your butt—*almost half a pound of fat*—see how that fits! The problem is—the label doesn't tell you directly that the whole bag has 1,500 Calories in it. It says, "150 Calories per serving," and then somewhere else, in small print, it mentions that *oh, by the way*, there are ten servings *in this teensy, tiny bag* and one serving equals one ounce (about 11 chips). Eleven chips—*come on!* That's a mouthful that doesn't even get me to the end of the opening kickoff.

One evening a few years ago, Sue complained about how often she was filling up the cereal jar, which was a one-and-a-half-gallon, lidded, clear glass container sitting on the countertop next to our appliance garage. Sue would mix cereal, nuts, and dried fruit in it for me so I could get off to the salt mine that much quicker every day, so as to better support her habits.

"Exactly how much cereal do you eat in the morning?" she asked.

"A bowlful," I answered—*what a ridiculous question.*

"Do you know how many servings are in a 'bowlful'?"

At this I paused. I thought of the 2.5 servings in a bottle of Gatorade. *Uh-oh.* "Not exactly."

"Well, maybe you should measure it out."

"Yeah, you're right, baby." *Of course she was.* And all the while I was thinking of finding a bigger bowl, because by the time I added my strawberries there wasn't enough room for the skim milk.

The next morning I checked the label. One cup per serving with one-half cup of skim milk added up to 230 Calories. Okay—*deep breath*—I got my bowl and filled it up to the customary level half an inch from the top. I took the one-cup scoop and emptied three servings, plus, back into the jar. *Shee-it!* I looked up the incidentals: ¼ cup of almonds (210 Calories), ¼ cup of dried cherries (80 Calories), one sliced banana (100 Calories). And did I mention that I love fruit? On my way out the door every morning I would grab a peach, apple, or plum, sometimes two (100 Calories), depending on the season. So, every morning, before 0730 I would have 230 times three, plus 210 plus 80 plus 100 plus 100+, or a minimum of 1,180 Calories under my belt and on my ass, given my propensity for an even split between android and gynoid obesity.

Fourth Principle of the Diet Theory of Everything

If it's good enough for you, it's good enough for the rest of your family.

This is easy for us because we are only a family of two. We have touched upon the endemic problem of obesity and the rising prevalence of obesity in children. If a low-fat, low glycemic index–carbohydrate, high-fiber diet is healthy and good for you, why would you want to pick up a high-fat, high glycemic index, low-fiber meal for the kids on your way home from work? The refined carbohydrates of white bread and French fries are the equivalent of table sugar, and all those fat grams are cumulative for the little guy or little gal over the course of their childhood. The only good thing about an order of fries for a toddler is that half of them end up on the floor.

I am not talking about suffering for the rest of your life on a sterile diet of rice cakes, celery stalks, and tuna out of a can. I am talking about gourmet meals, romantic evenings out, snacks, and even fast food on occasion. It is neither hard nor unpleasant. It is easier to prepare one meal rather than two, and what greater gift can you give your children than an appreciation for a healthy, wholesome diet and way of life that will become second nature for them? It may not be as obvious as piano lessons or a college education, but I feel that it is, at the very least, just as important. Why is it that we are more concerned with our children's orthodontic care, athletic endeavors, and sore throats rather than with their diet that impacts all of their precious little walks of life?

I understand that meal preparation takes time and is inconvenient. I realize that most families depend upon two incomes in which both spouses work, and that the single parent is overburdened with demands upon their time such that fast food is a convenience and seemingly a necessity all too often. Despite that, there are ways to cope with the crush of time for the evening meal.

Crock-Pot cooking is one solution. The main dish slowly cooks all day and is ready when you come home; then all you need to do is throw together a few sides, such as whole wheat pasta, frozen or fresh vegetables, a salad, and a squash or sweet potato. Our family has developed quite the fondness for sweet potato fries. Sue slices up a sweet potato and puts the "fries" in a zip-lock bag with a bit of olive oil, one teaspoon of Cajun seasoning, one teaspoon of paprika, and then she shakes it up and bakes them on a shallow pan for 25 minutes at 425 degrees.

We eat quite a bit of fish and chicken as our protein sources. Our meals can be quickly prepared from frozen chicken breasts or fish fillets, taken out of the freezer the night before, or defrosted in the microwave if I forgot to comply with Sue's frequent nighttime directive to take something out for dinner.

This is the new millennium. We have convection ovens, microwaves with different buttons for different foods, timed ovens, George Foreman grills, gas bar-beques, canned foods, and freezers. We can cook mul-tiple portions on the weekends and freeze them for the following weekdays. There really is no excuse; all that is required is a little bit of planning, free will, and positive action.

An example of what not to do

Sarah had a BMI of 29, or just under obese (high health risk). She saw her physician, who prescribed an appetite suppressant (phentermine) and recommended a weight-watcher program. Sarah was particularly motivated as she was looking forward to a twenty-year class reunion, three months away, where she anticipated running into an old flame. She decided to put herself on a Very Low Calorie Diet of less than a thousand Calories a day. The plan was to go from 185 lb. (BMI 29) to 146 lb. (BMI 23) as quickly as pos-sible. Sarah was happy to discover that she loved Thai soup, because it wasn't expensive, it was quick, and, best of all, it was on the way home from work, right next to a McDonald's. She would phone her order in, "I'd like one bowl of Tom Yam Spicy Shrimp and one cup of stir-fry vegetables, please," which amounted to a total of 260 Calories. Within minutes of placing her order, she'd take a right, out of the drive-way of the bank where she worked, stop by the "Be Thai and Stay Skinny Restaurant" to pick up her order; halfway down the block she'd turn right again, into the McDonald's drive-through for a Happy Meal for the kid strapped in the back—exit right, and, homeward bound.

Sarah didn't keep much food around in the house in the way of fresh fruits or vegetables. She didn't have much time to cook for herself or for her child, so most of their meals were fast-food drive-thru's. Sarah ate her food and her son ate his. Did I mention that Sarah hated exercise? She didn't have any time for it anyway, given the demands of her TV programs; therefore, her entire caloric deficit needed to come from a dietary restriction.

The pounds melted off. The slinky, size 12 dress fit like a glove and Sarah looked great in the dress, although at the hotel swimming pool the evening before the reunion she did find the Jello-like wiggle in her upper arms some-what disconcerting. How many evenings after the reunion do you think Sarah kept having hot and sour soup? Zero. Two months later Sarah was back in her larger sizes, with her slinky dress shoved, forgotten, to the back of the closet.

My transitioning to a state of awareness

I benefited directly from Sue's disciplined approach to her diet. Almost three years ago, sometime after that morning I couldn't find the scale in our bathroom, I started noticing things. A slick, black, digital scale appeared on our center island, and a small calorie-counter booklet manifested itself in the kitchen computer hutch. Sue was spending a lot of time looking up recipes online and ordered *The South Beach Diet Cookbook*. Boxes of meal replacement bars of 210 and 240 Calories and snack bars of 110 and 140 Calories were purchased and unpacked into a large bowl in the kitchen. She had resigned from an online Weight Watchers program a few weeks earlier and said something to the effect that she would *do it her damn self.*

I was amazed at the smallness of her portion size and would routinely eat three portions to her one. Although the size of her entrée looked small to me, the salad did not, and we always had a side of squash, brown rice or sweet potatoes, as well as a cooked vegetable such as brussels sprouts, asparagus, broccoli, or cauliflower. The entrées that we ate were incredible: Gingered Salmon, Grilled Mahi-Mahi with fruit-bean salsa, Peanut Chicken, Buffalo Pizza w/Turkey Pepperoni. Sue made sugar-free desserts and substituted applesauce for cooking oil. She made them in individual servings so that I could not cut my own piece—we had little tins of apple and cherry pie (sugar-free filling) with crust only on the top, and Jello-cake on which we'd put low fat or fat-free whipped topping. I had dessert every night.

During this time, Sue did not pressure me to cut back on my caloric intake, and although I generally avoided sweets at work most of the time, I still couldn't resist one or two every now and then. I ate breakfast, a hearty lunch, and my two-to-three-portion-sized dinner with a low-calorie dessert just about every evening. I'd grab a meal bar for a morning or afternoon snack and would usually have an apple from the doctors' lounge sometime during the day.

I exercised four times a week for a total of three to four hours. This consisted of running (summertime), swimming, riding an elliptical trainer, and lifting weights in my basement. I exercised more if I felt guilty for eating half a pizza in the staff lounge over lunch or if I went crazy at a restaurant and ate three baskets of white bread. Sometimes I would ride the elliptical trainer an extra half hour in *anticipation* of overeating.

I was a big one for weighing myself daily, and periodically throughout the day if I was feeling particularly skinny, which I rarely was, but I always had hope. I would weigh myself after a workout or a healthy number two, and occasionally several times in a row because I didn't think the scale was right the first time.

Prior to the 2004 Door County Triathlon (sprint-distance—0.25-mile swim, 12-mile bike, 3-mile run) I weighed 239 lb. I had been as low as 229 in the few weeks before but then company came and I started carbo-loading because that's what I read about in my triathlete books and magazines. *I needed those carbohydrates.* The problem was that I was only doing a sprint-distance race, and sprinkled in between all those carbohydrates were several pieces of gourmet cheesecake, sugar cookies, homemade bread, and the usual three square meals a day, which were especially scrumptious because of our visiting relatives. My heart sank the morning of the race when the red digital readout blinked 239...239...239. It didn't change the second or third time I weighed myself either.

Three years ago, the morning of my second annual sprint-distance triathlon, the readout told me I was 229 lb. By the end of the triathlon I was probably 225 lb. It was hotter than Hades, with a heat index over 100 degrees, and the medical tent was full of triathletes with IV's and others getting ice baths. Sue took a picture of me standing under the "Door County Triathlon" sign and I looked great. I was 44 years old and, hands down, in the best shape of my life. I shot Sue a "Schwarzenegger" pose, and a reporter from the paper came up and talked to me. I felt like I was twenty years old again. Alas, the zenith of my corporeal existence was only transient. One hour after crossing the finish line, I was home in the kitchen devouring a plate of frosted sugar cookies I found on the center island that my visiting niece and nephew had somehow overlooked. And since I had taken the week off to recover from my *sprint-distance* triathlon I had stopped exercising but didn't stop eating. By the following Sunday my "Spartan-ness" had dissipated like a morning fog dispersed by a stiff wind.

A few months later, the holidays hit; the same relatives came back. I found myself in competition with my sister-in-law for the last pieces of rum cake and Brandy Alexander cheesecake and with my niece, nephew, and granddaughter for the frosted sugar cookies. By early January, my 38s were getting uncomfortably tight and I was missing the size 40s I had donated to Goodwill in a fit of optimism.

February found me back in my XXX scrubs. By this point in time, Sue had been on her self-designed diet for about eight months, and I don't know how much she weighed or how much weight she had lost—*even she didn't know how much she weighed*—but she looked great. I was happy for Sue; at the same time I was puzzled by my lack of weight loss, as I had increased my exercise from four hours a week to five. I had also cut out sweets at work and only had a low calorie dessert every *other* night.

So I said to her one night after supper, halfway through dessert, "I don't get it. I exercise like I'm

possessed, eat sensibly, and just can't lose weight." I
waited for a sympathetic reply; maybe a hug or kiss, or a
tender touch, but she only said, "You eat too much."

"I must have a tumor or something—it just isn't
natural."

"Your portion size is huge. You have a dessert every
night and that is 180 Calories, without the whipped
cream, and you don't exercise *that much*." She said this
not at all sympathetically.

"If you want to lose weight, just say the word and
I'll take you down. I'll take you waaay down." She followed her promise with a sinister chuckle that caused
the hair on my arms to stand up. It was a night or two
later that she commented on the rapid diminishment
of the cereal jar. Thus began the process of my gradual
enlightenment.

The next morning was a Wednesday. For the first time
in years I weighed myself just once that day—and every
week thereafter. I weighed 260 lb.—a gain of 35 lb. from
my triathlon weight, seven months previously—kind of
like a Holiday gift to myself.

Food intake on a typical day pre-enlightenment

Calorie counting

Meal	Description	Calories
Breakfast	Kashi Go Lean with almonds, dried cherries, and blueberries, with sliced strawberries or banana, plus an apple on the way to work	1,200
Morning snack	Rum cake—my medical assistant, Linda, brought this in to work because I had brought some last Christmas and she knew I was fond of it. She had a piece sitting on my desk	600

Meal	Description	Calories
Lunch	A drug rep brought in pizza—I eat four pieces of a deep pan Meat Lover's	340 × 4 = 1,360
Afternoon snack	I'm feeling guilty so I just have an apple	100
Supper	Sue makes a ginger-baked salmon on whole grain rice of which I have three servings (690). Incidentals are squash (½), which I doctor up with butter and brown sugar and honey, *yummy!* (250), Brussels sprouts (100), salad with light dressing (60), Michelob Ultra (95), Sue's low calorie dessert w/ whipped cream (200)	1,165
Evening snack	Pear (95), apple (70)	165
Total count for day		4,820

Holy buckets! Sue's not impressed. She says she's got a headache.

A usual period of exercise would be forty minutes on the elliptical trainer that tells me I burned 800 Calories. At this point in my life, size forty, I am about 260 lb; my daily requirement for maintenance is 260 lb. × 11 Calories per pound, which equals 2,860 Calories per day. If I subtract this and the 800 Calories for the exercise in my otherwise sedentary life of a surgeon I am left with a 1,160-Calorie positive energy balance, which adds up in three short days to a pound of stored energy in my rapidly expanding fat cells. Granted, the rum cake was a little rich, I obviously don't eat that every day, but substitute a couple of cookies or lemon bars or glazed donuts— even a midget-sized granola bar has 140 Calories. Clearly,

I don't eat pizza every day either, but a serving of meat loaf, baked French fries, buttered vegetables, and a piece of fruit from the cafeteria are probably not much less.

Food intake on a typical day post-enlightenment

Calorie counting

Meal	Description	Calories
Breakfast	Kashi Go Lean with dried cherries, apple (70)	390
Morning snack	Snack bar	140
Lunch	I smelled pizza in the hallway to the lounge—didn't even open the door. Chicken thigh/drumstick (skinless, no breading) (185) and vegetables (80), whole wheat hard roll without butter—I'm a sucker for bread (120), apple (70) from the cafeteria	455
Afternoon snack	Snack bar	140
Supper	Turkey thigh cooked in a slow roaster pot all day long (235), baked Cajun sweet potato fries (70), salad (60), asparagus spears (30), individual apple pie with whipped cream (200)	595
Evening snack	Apple (70), sugar-free strawberry popsicle with real fruit, mmm (35)	105
Total count for day		*1,825*

Sue is verily impressed. She can't wipe the smile off her face. I'm feeling lucky. Assuming the same variables as the pre-enlightened state, except skipping the exercise because I had such a hard day dieting, gives us 1,830 – 2,750 = –920 Calories, or a daily *thermodynamicu-*

lar deficit of 920 Calories, which equals one pound of fat from my shriveling adipocytes every 3.8 days. Adding in the exercise would almost double the deficit. I think you can tell from the above daily record that I didn't suffer unduly. I did deprive myself of the camaraderie in the staff lounge at lunchtime, but I am sure that everyone got by just fine without me.

Macronutrient recommendations

As I have said, the bottom line is that you can eat whatever you want, as long as it is within your calculated daily caloric need. The only thing you have to do is eat the obligatory protein (0.8 g/kg), which is only sixteen ounces for a 300-pounder. If you skimp too much on your protein, you'll get a big belly from ascites (intra-abdominal fluid) secondary to kwashiorkor (protein-deficient) malnutrition, and that would mess up your measurements.

Snickers bar diet

How about a Snickers bar diet? That sounds good to me. I *love* Snickers bars. After all, it is the world's most popular candy bar, with over two billion dollars in annual sales. We better stick to the regular candy bar, as opposed to the Snickers pie with over 1,250 Calories per slice in fat and sugar alone. We'll also avoid the deep-fried Snickers at the fairgrounds; instead, we'll carry our own personal supply. Now let's do the math. We'll even throw in a multivitamin pill for the trace elements and a vitamin C so we don't get scurvy and lose all our teeth, like the poor bastards who rounded Cape Horn in a wooden sailboat, *before* James Lind *deduced* that all you needed to do was suck on a lemon wedge every other day.

Snickers bar (2.07 oz.)
values from published nutritional label

Carbohydrate	36 g
Protein	4 g
Fat	14 g
Fiber	1 g
Calories	280
Vitamins	A (2 percent DV)
	Calcium (4 percent DV)
	Iron (4 percent DV)

At a targeted weight of 220 lb, as we have previously determined, I have a caloric requirement of 2,420 Calories per day. Now let's divide this by 280 and I get 8.6 Snickers bars per day. I'll be generous and round this up to 9 Snickers bars per day for a total caloric intake of 2,520 Calories per day.

Now we'll calculate my macronutrients:

Carbohydrate	36 g – 1 g fiber = 35 g
	35 g × 3.8 = 133 Calories*
Protein	4 g × 4 = 16 Calories
Fat	14 g × 9.3 = 130 Calories†

* Calculated at 3.8 Cal/g. By convention, this is rounded up to 4 Cal/g.

† Calculated at 9.3 Cal/g. By convention, this is rounded down to 9 Cal/g.

Carbohydrate:protein:fat ratio = 48:6:46.

The Snickers bar diet is like a *reverse* Atkins, before our modifications.

Since I am only interested in the protein content in regard to the above, I calculate the daily protein intake by multiplying the four grams per bar by nine bars, which gives me a total of 36 g. At 220 lb., I need 80 grams for the day—uh-oh, looks like big-belly time for me, unless I supplement the Snickers bar diet with some 100 percent, chocolate-flavored whey protein. At 23 g per scoop, it looks like I'll need two scoops for a total of 82 g of protein per day, which will give me a little safety margin. *Hold on*—110 Calories per scoop—looks like we'd better lose a Snickers bar and its attendant 4 g of protein—so 32 g (eight Snickers bars) + 46 g (whey) = 78 g of daily protein. *Whoops*—there goes my safety margin, but, heck, that's close enough.

To round out my Snickers bar diet, I'd better add some fiber to ease the daily business. I like Citrucel, sugar free. The daily fiber requirement for an adult male is 38 g (30 g for a female). Given that I already have accounted for eight grams from the eight Snickers bars, I only need 31 g more. At 2 g per scoop that means I'll need 15 scoops throughout the day, which is good because it means I'll drink plenty of water. Aren't we supposed to drink eight glasses of water a day? And all that fiber will help take the edge off my hunger that I am sure to have, secondary to the rebounding hypoglycemic effect of the multiple insulin surges. *Oh no!!!* I just noticed that each dose sugar-free Citrucel has 24 Calories of maltodextrin (sugar alcohol). This means that I need 360 (15 × 24) Calories of Citrucel—looks like I'll need to lose a couple of more Snickers bars, add a scoop of whey powder, and an extra scoop of Citrucel.

After all of this fine-tuning, the Snickers bar diet looks like this:

Meal	Description	Calories
Breakfast	2 Snickers bars (560) and 10 scoops of Citrucel in 10 glasses of water, since this is the most important meal of the day (240), 1 scoop whey (110)	910
Morning snack	1 Snickers bar (280)	280
Lunch	1 Snickers bar (280), 1 scoop Citrucel in 1 glass of water (24), 1 scoop whey (110)	414
Afternoon snack	2 scoops Citrucel in 2 glasses of water (48)—*mmmm…yummy*	48
Supper	2 Snickers bars (560), 1 scoop Citrucel in 1 glass of water (24), 1 scoop whey (110)	694
Evening snack	2 scoops Citrucel in 2 glasses of water (48)	48
Other	Multivitamin tablet (negligible), vitamin C (negligible)	0
Total count for day		2,394

Breakdown of macronutrients

Carbohydrate	213 g =	852 Calories
including sugar alcohol		384 Calories
Total carbohydrate	=	1,236 Calories
Protein	93 g =	372 Calories
Fat	88.5 g =	796 Calories

Taken in proportion to my daily requirement of 2,400 Cal, the ratio of carbohydrate:protein:fat is 52:16:33.

Notice anything? This ratio is only three percentage points off of what the Heart Healthy Diet recommends, the diet that has been trumpeted by governmental health institutions for the past fifty-plus years—a Snickers bar diet equivalent. Nonetheless, this is a viable diet. You could cross the Atlantic on this and not lose your teeth or get a swollen belly. I couldn't do it. I ate ten Snickers bars in one day while doing a golf marathon, in addition to breakfast, lunch, and dinner, and I was still hungry.

Well, this was a fun exercise, and it does demonstrate that the general public has been snookered—*snickered?*—for several decades in regard to dietary recommendations. There have been recent studies that have produced results counter to the long-held belief that a low-fat diet is much more important than a lower-carbohydrate diet. This is something that deserves its own chapter, so keep reading.

More appropriate macronutrient recommendations

Carbohydrate

It is not important to count carbohydrates, specifically, since we are primarily interested in the energy content. In restricting yourself to a certain amount of calories, which includes a more generous portion of protein, you will, by default, consume a smaller proportion of carbohydrates in an appropriate ratio. Your choice of carbohydrates should, however, be limited to lower glycemic index sources, such as whole grains, pasta, most fruits and vegetables, sweet potatoes, and yams. You need to avoid the high glycemic index sources found in the refined sugars and starches, like white potatoes, white rice, corn, white bread, and Snickers bars.

Your calorie-counter book should have a list of low glycemic index foods; also, there is a plethora of websites with online databases (www.glycemicindex.com). Substitute Splenda for sugar in cooking and use other artificial sweeteners* as needed.

Protein

On a calorie-restricted diet you must, at the minimum, pay homage to your minimum daily protein requirement of 0.8 g/kg/day. It shouldn't be that hard to hit, especially for the carnivorous. In reality, the ideal is to exceed the minimum requirement such that the proportion of protein as a total of your daily caloric requirement is higher. I have mentioned this earlier, but I look for foods with almost as much protein (in grams) as net carbohydrates (in grams). An added benefit of protein is its satiety effect (fat also causes satiety).

If you prefer cereal for breakfast, find one that is high in fiber and protein, such as Kashi Go Lean, which has 9 g of protein in one serving, and unless you eat your cereal dry, you'll get another 5 g in the ½ cup of skim milk that accompanies it. One large egg, or the equivalent lower-fat egg substitute, has 6 g of protein; 75 Calories for the egg and 30 for the egg substitute. Eight ounces of low-fat yogurt holds 12 g of protein at the cost of 208 Calories.

Unless your target weight is 300 lb., which would mean that you're seven feet tall, your protein requirement is likely much less than a chicken a day. By the end of breakfast, with a single serving of cereal at a caloric cost of 240 Calories, you would have met 25 percent of your daily need at a weight of 175 lb. You will probably have an equivalent amount for lunch, and don't forget the snacks—a low calorie snack bar could have as much

---

* There is some recent debate about the benignity of artificial sweeteners, which is discussed more completely in a later chapter.

as 10 g of protein. By the time you get to supper, which is most likely the largest protein meal of the day, you'll be just fine. Most likely, you will comfortably exceed your protein requirement, and that is a good thing because of the DIT that we reviewed earlier. The caloric expense of digesting all that healthy food negates the total caloric value by approximately 10–20 percent—*finally, something for nothing.*

High-fat protein sources should be avoided in general. If you do consume these sources, you will have to eat less, as the caloric cost is subtracted from your daily requirement. Red meat equivalents such as bison, buffalo, elk, emu, ostrich, and venison are excellent, low-fat sources of protein but are about twice as expensive. Extra-lean ground beef and lean beefsteaks are just fine as a source of protein. My family's primary animal protein sources are fish, poultry, and bison, when we find it. I would have made a very good Native American.

Fat

Since you won't be eating high-fat foods on a regular basis, this shouldn't be a problem. If you eat too much fat, it will be reflected as a large percentage of your daily caloric allotment and you won't be eating as much food, and that will get tiresome after a while, as long as you maintain your course. This means no pizza (unless it's made with a whole wheat crust, low-fat cheese, and turkey pepperoni or low fat meat), no burger joints, a careful selection of an entrée when eating out, no Doritos, no ice cream. I'll let you figure out the rest by using your calorie-counter database.

Use margarine or light butter and, when cooking, use extra virgin olive oil whenever you can. Resources available online, such as recipe databases, food diaries, and calorie counters, will be of great benefit. There are several high-quality, low-calorie cookbooks that cover a wide range of tastes and ingredients. They offer great tips, such as substituting *no sugar added* applesauce for cooking oil and low-fat yogurt for sour cream.

The primary fat to avoid is saturated fat that is a solid at room temperature, like the white fat in hamburger or the marbling of a rib eye. Carbon atoms in saturated fat share electrons with hydrogen atoms rather than another carbon atom, and it is therefore said to be hydrogenated, or saturated (with hydrogen). In contrast, the unsaturated fats have carbon atoms that do not share electrons with hydrogen and, therefore, *are not* saturated with hydrogen. They are considered good fats and should compose a healthy majority of your daily fat intake. These fats are liquids at room temperature: olive, canola, soy, flax, and walnut oils are all examples. The omega-3 fatty acids are polyunsaturated fats in which several studies have demonstrated positive health benefits such as improvement in cardiovascular disease, decrease in cholesterol levels and a possible anti-cancer effect. They are essential fatty acids, which means that the body cannot synthesize them. Foods rich in omega-3 fatty acids include oily fishes such as salmon, herring and sardines, and plant sources such as flax and sesame seeds, and walnuts.

chapter thirteen

Eating out

ATING OUT IS A lot easier than it used to be. Some restaurants have lighter fare or low-calorie menus. A good fast-food alternative is a Subway turkey/ham with half the cheese or no cheese— Sue and Jessie (our daughter) like the six-inch veggie sub on whole wheat with light mayo. It is possible to select an entrée from a menu that will do no harm, but beware of cream-based sauces and cheeses. For instance, one evening Sue and I went out to eat at Applebee's and in order to blunt the sharp edge of my hunger, I ordered a Veggie Patch Pizza as an appetizer. I ate four of the six pieces. Imagine my surprise when Sue looked it up in our calorie counter upon arriving home (it wasn't listed on the menu) and told me it was 150 Calories per serving, of which I had four (600 Cal)! *Torpedoed again, and it sounded so healthy.*

Then there are those times when you might be celebrating something special, like my daughter's ex-boyfriend's birthday, and just say *what the hell.*

Casablanca is a Middle Eastern restaurant in downtown Milwaukee where Sue and I took Jessica, and her friend Tom, to celebrate his birthday.

"Say there, Tom, why don't you be a sport and pass me the pita bread." There were two baskets of bread on the table, but I had already exhausted the one closest to my end. "Anybody want the rest of that hummus?" After an obligatory pause, like at a stop sign when nobody's looking, I scraped the plate clean and heaped the chickpea stuff on my flatbread—it's a vegetable, I reassured myself, forgetting my Veggie Patch Pizza lesson.

I was crazy hungry by the time we sat down to eat. I had been depriving myself all day, and by depriving myself I mean to say *skipping lunch*. For breakfast I had my typical bowl of Kashi cereal, doctored up with dried cherries and a few nuts, I think almonds, and topped off with a freshly sliced banana (pre-enlightenment).

We had reservations for six p.m. The only speed bump was a new mall on the north side of Milwaukee that the girls wanted to stop at—just for a few minutes, they said. Ravenous as I was, my fantasy was that we'd arrive half an hour early at the restaurant to warm up with a few drinks and the Middle Eastern equivalent of chicken wings before dinner. My only hope, now that a new mall loomed on the horizon, was that I'd find a health food store passing out samples of muscle milk.

Jessie must have picked up on my anxiety about not making it to the restaurant on time, because from the backseat I heard her reassuring voice, "No problem, Dad. I know this place like the back of my hand. We only need five minutes to get to Casablanca." Still doubtful, I pulled off the comfortable familiarity of I-43 into congested five o'clock traffic and headed towards the mall.

Turns out it was an outdoor mall, but a very nice one, other than the twenty-degree-below windchill factor on that crisp February evening. As we strolled along, facing into a robust north wind, Sue asked Tom, "Tom, where's your coat?"

"Didn't bring it," he said, being a man of few words.

"I told him to bring his coat but he said, 'What the hell do I need a coat for. We're just going to dinner.'" Jessie said this in the tone of voice known to man since at least the Pleistocene epoch.

Thinking to spare Tom from the cold and further assaults on his ego, I said, "Hey, let's check out this store." The frozen breath from my words was swept away by the door as I pulled it open and stepped to the side, allowing the blast of warmth from inside to rush over Tom.

We all entered The Chair Store, which sounded interesting. It was an ergonomic chair store. In no time at all the store owner, named Joe, had me fitted in a high-backed leather office chair that I initially thought was a barber chair because it had an orthotic look to it, like a pair of big boxy shoes. His wife, Betty, had Sue stretched out and supine on an electric massage table. Tom and Jessie didn't garner much initial attention, I suppose because they looked less affluent than Sue and me. Not being in the mood to plunk down three thousand dollars for an office chair, even if an ergonomic one, I strolled around the store.

"Do you suffer from any chronic back pain, Shaun?" Joe asked.

"Not really, Joe. We're all pretty healthy. No major aches and pains." Joe, a little disappointed, refocused on Sue, still in the horizontal position on the Shiatsu massage table.

"How much does this table run, Joe?" Sue asked. My ears perked up.

"That's $1,999.00," he said, which was the same price for the zero-gravity chair Jessie had just asked him about. Joe chuckled. "Pretty much everything in the store is $1,999.00." *Except the office chair*, I wanted to add.

"Honey, you got to try this." I looked at my watch— five thirty.

"Okay." I kicked off my shoes and assumed the position. I didn't feel anything at first because the rollers were behind my knees. Then, fairly abruptly, I felt these steel balls and other metal parts moving up behind my thighs. They were hard and demanded that I be relaxed and flexible, which I definitely wasn't, worried as I was about missing our reservation. My jeans, relaxed-fit 38-waist, were kind of tight, which further increased my discomfiture because I felt like everyone was checking out my unit. The metal or wood rollers, or whatever they were, hurt as they pushed into my unyielding flesh. The mechanical masseuse bumped and grinded its way up my spine. I arched my back, grimaced, and then I heard a bone crack. "My sternum cracked." I wiggled my shoulders, checking for pain. "I think I popped a wire." Joe looked at me, a smile frozen on his face. I could see a rim of white over the top of his irises. We doctors call that "lid lag;" it is a sign of anxiety, or thyrotoxicosis, which is due to an elevated thyroid hormone. I doubted that Joe was thyrotoxic.

"Are you okay?" he asked me.

"Yeah, I'm fine." As an afterthought I added, "I think," just in case I really wasn't. A vision of dollar signs ran through my head, or at least a vision of a free ergonomic office chair with tufted leather, padded arms, and a cherry wood base.

"He had open heart surgery a few years ago," Sue offered by way of an explanation. Joe nodded sympathetically and dabbed his forehead with a handkerchief. He seemed puzzled—I suppose from my reassurance of our robust health mere seconds earlier.

I checked my watch—five thirty-five. "Thanks for your time, Joe. We have to leave for dinner." Joe was overjoyed with our departure. He held the door open for us as we left, hoping, I am sure, to never set eyes upon us again. Jessie drove from the mall since she knew where she was going, except that she didn't; or else we experienced a quantum time contraction, because it took us twenty-five minutes to cover a reportedly five-minute distance.

Casablanca, the town, is in Morocco; and Casablanca, the restaurant, was consistent with the desert theme. There was a huge mural of sand dunes, with an oasis and camel in the background, on one wall. The lighting was subdued. Hidden in the shadows of one corner was a small elevated stage for belly dancing on Friday nights and I felt sorry for it being a Saturday. I closed my eyes…

I imagine a shapely, dark-skinned woman with purple-black eyes, like Elizabeth Taylor in Antony *and* Cleopatra, *moving sinuously to the intoxicating sound of ancient Egyptian music. She teases me with the soft tinkle of finger cymbals, and as she moves closer, the sweet scent of jasmine brushes against my face and I can see the lustrous sparkle of a ruby in her navel, promising of further treasures of the Arabian night.*

"Shaun…Shaun."

"Hunh? Oh, I'm not sure what I'm having yet." My vision of Elizabeth Taylor popped like a beautiful iridescent soap bubble hitting the pavement and was replaced by my wife's visage immediately to my right.

"What are you talking about? I just wanted to know if you saw the hookah pipes on the wall when we came in."

"Uh, no, must have missed 'em."

"Well, maybe we can try one after supper."

"Yeah, we'll see," which translated means, no, we won't. "Doesn't that cause cancer?"

After twenty years of holy matrimony my beloved had no need of an interpreter, and as she wasn't sure about the cancer thing herself, she must have decided to let it pass because she refocused on Jessie across the table. This freed me up to focus on Tom, who I figured would need a lot of focusing anyway.

A young lady with chocolate eyes and a silky voice, looking strangely like my imaginary belly dancer, sans ruby, stopped by our table. "May I get you anything to drink?" I looked into her face and thought of the desert, harems, and Arabian nights.

"I'll take a Miller Lite," said Tom.

The girls both decided on the rose lemonade. "I'll try that rose lemonade, too, please." *What the hell.*

Within minutes, Tom was sucking down a tall frosty while I was quaffing vase water, or what I imagined vase water would taste like. The girls seemed to like it so much that I pushed my glass their way and waited patiently for the return of our slippered servant girl.

In no time at all, our desert beauty had supplied us with three appetizers, baskets of bread, and more Miller Lite. I inhaled two cabbage rolls with rice and meat (200), four tablespoons of baba ghanouj (eggplant) (140), a half cup of hummus (210); since I had to put all that spread on something, I found that the five pieces of pita bread served quite nicely (759). By the time the entrée came, shawarma (spit roast beef) (700), the edge was gone, and we all had a grand time. For dessert, we decided to forgo the colorful hookah pipes and had baklava instead (300). I didn't share. With beverages included, my caloric intake for dinner was 2,500 Calories. This amounted to my entire daily requirement *just for dinner*. And this isn't bad, considering the volume of food I ate. If you're going to overindulge, I'd suggest Middle Eastern anytime—but especially on Friday nights.

What about the energy costs of a few other more common meals out on the town?

Tell you what: I'm in the mood for a margarita and chips. *How about a Mexican dinner?*

Item	Calories
Chimichangas, beef, 5 oz. × 2	800
Sour cream, 2 Tbsp	60
Refried beans, ¾ cup	160
Spanish rice, 4 oz.	160
Tortilla chips, 1 basket	1,000
Guacamole, 1 oz.	120
Margarita (small)	156
Flan, 5.5 oz.	305
Total	2,761

You know, I just don't have any time today; I'll just stop by Culver's drive-through on my way home from work.

Item	Calories
Bacon Deluxe ButterBurger	765
Cheese curds	710
Turtle sundae	1,245
Coke	210
Total	2,930

Culture of fat

We live in a culture of fat—fast food, fatty food, large portions, convenience, taste—all in the name of pleasuring the id—*Id wants, Id gets*. It is a market-driven system, which isn't a bad thing, because, if enough people change, then the market will change as well. Wouldn't it be nice if there were a breakdown of the carbohydrate, protein, fat, and caloric content of every meal selection? There isn't; and, until there is, you will need to figure it out on your own.

If everyone understood the spirit of my book and changed their lifestyles accordingly, much else would change as well. What would happen to all the fast-food hamburger joints, the pizza industry, the candy bar business, and the National Association of Glazed Donuts and Sugar Cookies? Burger King, McDonald's, Taco Bell, Taco John's, Wendy's, Culver's, and Pizza Hut: all of these places are successful because of the choices we make. The cost seems reasonable; the food is convenient and tastes good, and the kids desperately need the enticing paraphernalia that comes with their high-fat burger on white bread, deep-fried white potato fries, and 180-Calorie soda pop.

The entire food industry would be forced to change, because business people want to make money, which is a good thing, not an evil thing—that is called capitalism. In a relatively short time, the supply of healthier choices would rise to meet the demand; and then we would be able to drive up to McDonald's and order a buffalo burger on whole wheat, baked sweet potato fries, a side of asparagus seasoned with a touch of extra virgin olive oil, salt and pepper, and a Diet Coke to go. We would be able to take the kids to Pizza Hut for a whole wheat crust pizza with turkey pepperoni and low-fat cheese. Mexican restaurants would have whole wheat, baked chips and salsa, and tacos with extra-lean ground chuck.

But the food industry will not change *first*. Our culture of fat will chug along, like it always has, until you change. There is not the impetus for them to change first—that would be too expensive. When the Atkins diet was all the rage and half the people you passed on the street were in the induction phase, you can be sure that the bread industry felt the pinch, because soon thereafter loaves of whole wheat bread, sliced thin and labeled as low-carbohydrate, magically appeared on the grocery store shelves. You couldn't turn a corner in a grocery store without stumbling over a stack of a low-carb this or low-carb that, and sandwiched between every chip and soda aisle was an end cap of pork rinds.

Meal replacement bars, high in protein and fiber and not loaded with sugar, have become ubiquitous, replacing the conventional candy bar as a source of nourishment. Entrepreneurs have invented snack and energy bars in kitchens and shipped them out of their garages before becoming wildly successful international companies. What the people want, the people get, eventually; but *the people have to want it first*. That is the America we live in. Isn't it wonderful?

chapter fourteen

The holidays

HAVE UNDONE IN SIX weeks what took me an entire year to accomplish. For some reason, during Thanksgiving and Christmas, anything goes. It's like a vacation—a vacation from common sense. Thanksgiving 2003 is a sad example of this. It's not only Thanksgiving Day and Christmas Day; it's the days before and the days after, especially those days with company. We typically will have two to three families with us over the course of the holidays, and obviously they are not there just for Christmas, or just for Thanksgiving, because no one would drive 500 miles to spend one day. We have, therefore, one gluttonous week around each of the Holidays—a week in which every day is a party.

Thanksgiving 2003

I was the first one up, other than my seven-year-old niece, who was watching the *101 Dalmatians* videotape that I had started for her. Brad would be by in half an hour and then he, my brother-in-law, son, and I were going scuba diving off of the northern tip of the peninsula. All of my scuba gear was in a relative state of entropy and I wanted to make sure that we had everything, but I knew that if I forgot something Brad would be sure to have an extra.

By the time I came back into the house, Sue had breakfast under way, and before we headed north, loaded up to the gills with underwater life-support systems, we, too, were loaded up to the gills with deer sausage, eggs, bacon and pancakes. My breakfast consisted of two links of sausage (200), two eggs (150), four strips of bacon (160), three pancakes (465) and a glass of orange juice (165). Sue was kind enough to pack several summer sausage and cheese sandwiches on buns with mayonnaise and a few bags of chips to ease the caloric burden of our diving.

Brad, who is a young friend of the family, and my son, Jason, had wet suits. My brother-in-law, Jimmy, and I had new dry suits, with pee valves installed the night before. Jimmy had brought with him a couple of condom catheters that he called Cuban wide-bands. He reassured me that they were watertight and would stay on all day. I installed it before we left the house, hoping it wouldn't hurt too much when it was time to take it off.

We were at the dive site an hour later, suited up and plugged into our pee valves (Jimmy and myself); Brad was last because of his affinity for redundancy, which I came to appreciate more the following year. Thirty minutes after pulling up to the beach we were eighty feet down and my bladder told me it was time. In the past when diving in a wet suit, I wouldn't drink at all because I didn't like the thought of swimming in piss, even if it was warm. This morning, however, was different. Secure in the capability of my Cuban wide-band and some inches of circumferential adhesive, I drank everything. I had a thermos of coffee, diet coke, orange juice, more of Brad's coffee—I was fearless. I could hardly wait to flood my pee-valve while underwater—I was looking forward to the illicit pleasure of actually relieving myself in a place not normal.

It was gorgeous. The visibility was at least 50 feet. I was bringing up the rear as we slowly moved along a steep slope of stone ledges and boulders. A rock bass looked at me, soon to be the only witness to my momentous event. I tried to relax my internal urethral sphincter, but I was a little nervous, what with it being my first time and all. Then, just as it had been hard, it was now suddenly easy—the tension left me, like a Kegel exercise in reverse. My lips stretched wide in a smile around the mouthpiece of my regulator. I imagined the rock bass smiling back. For a brief second there was the glorious pain of a distended bladder soon to be relieved, but then the floodgates opened, and I couldn't have stopped if I had wanted to. The hot football of urine behind my pubic bone felt heavy and good as I pushed. The pressurized stream of urine slammed into my Cuban wide-band and I moaned into the regulator as my vision blurred with the pupillary dilation accompanying my release.

The first sense of something amiss was a disconcerting warmth on the inside of my lower thigh, well below where I thought the tubing should be. A vision of an O-ring that I remembered coming with the tubing floated through my consciousness. *Damn. I knew it seemed too easy when I hooked it up.* Shortly thereafter, I felt the same warmth in my left foot, where I knew the tubing definitely was not.

By the time we stumbled out of the 42-degree water onto the stone beach, I couldn't feel my left leg. It was bluish-white and when I poked it curiously with my index finger, it felt like recently thawed steak. I could have cut a tenderloin from my upper thigh and not felt a thing. Urine was sloshing around inside the left leg of my dry suit and I smelled like a wet diaper. Of course, the boys made great sport of me over our lunch. I assuaged my embarrassment by hammering down two summer sausage buns (1,000) and five servings of Doritos (750) softened up by a couple of tall cold ones; Guinness (250).

We all know what afternoon and Thanksgiving means—football, beer, appetizers, and more beer. I can't remember who was playing, but I'm sure it was a good game. Little smokies in barbeque sauce (300), cheese, crackers, and sliced sausage (500), more Guinness (375), and chips with dip (600)—*rah, rah, rah, go, team, go*. We had a great time; after football we had dinner.

Since we had so many guests there was both turkey and ham. The side dishes were the staples of Thanksgiving dinners all over the nation: mashed potatoes and brown gravy, corn, cranberries, fruit salad, dressing; and as if that wasn't enough, Sue had also made pee-pee pasta (totally unrelated to the pee-valve), some creamy vegetable stuff with breading, and rice dressing. Just in case anyone choked on a turkey bone, she also had made three different kinds of bread, including my favorite, piña colada with shredded coconut.

As with every Thanksgiving, I had a turkey hind-quarter (235) as I prefer dark meat, but I also had a slice or two of white meat (200) because it's supposed to be better for you and it wasn't dried out yet. Naturally, the spiral-cut ham deserved my attention as well, one slice

(150). Potatoes and gravy (200), dressing (200), rice (250), corn (200), pee-pee pasta (300). I had one or two of everything, and in between all that I tucked one fourth of a two-pound loaf of piña colada bread in intermittent thick slices, picked up with each return trip to the center island (600).

All that food made me thirsty, but it was nothing a couple more tall cold ones couldn't handle (250). By the time dessert was served, I was stuffed. Do you think that stopped me? Of course not—I couldn't refuse a piece of cherry pie (500) from the Inn at Cedar Creek because I knew that if I didn't have one then, there wouldn't be any left later. The only reason I ate the piece of sour cream raisin pie (400) was because it was my all-time favorite.

I don't know where I found the room for two servings of pumpkin Bombay dessert (1,000) later in the evening while watching TV. I couldn't even get up, so I asked my niece, Morgan, to bring it to me. As soon as I swallowed the last spoonful of the cream cheese, graham-cracker, whipped-cream dessert, I felt awful. I didn't even want to think about it. By the next morning, I was digging into a tall stack of pancakes, absolutely ravenous.

Let's do the math. *Gulp*—9,300 Calories—and I'm sure I probably left something out—*oh, yeah, the turkey gizzards*, about another 100 Cal. Subtract a daily expenditure of 3,000 Calories and that leaves over six thousand excess Calories, or nearly two pounds of fat, *in one day*. Factor in a couple of days on either side of that, account for the three to ten holiday parties between Thanksgiving and Christmas, tack on Christmas and New Year's—and, *BAM!* I suddenly found myself sitting at my desk in a muumuu shirt, scratching the site of a future venous stasis ulcer on my edematous left ankle,

making a list of resolutions for the New Year, and thinking that maybe I'd need a motorized scooter to get my
groceries.

I was ill. I had violated the second deadly sin multiple
times in a most grievous fashion. I was not emotionally
healthy. I had no idea of the daily caloric requirement
for my gradually broadening bulk. I suffered from a distorted body image and thought that, since I was such a
"big guy," I needed more calories than everybody else.
Sue would refer to me intermittently as the "fat bastard,"
in reference to the obese, Scottish character played by
Mike Meyers in comedic skits on *Saturday Night Live*. I
was in my XXX scrubs more often than not, and one day
in the OR, halfway through a meal bar, I dramatically
pronounced, "It takes 4,000 Calories just for me to open
my eyes every morning." I was over a 1,000 Calories off,
and every three days that added up to a pound of fat.

After my annual inflationary period, my caloric intake would normalize, but only to a level of relative maintenance of my post-holiday expanded heft. My psychological set point was such that I was used to eating about
3,500–4,000 Calories a day, which covered my dietary
intake and a bit of exercise. I suspect this is where a lot of
overweight people reside. They are at an excess weight,
based on the foods that they are used to eating, and their
excess caloric intake maintains the excess weight, with
a tendency to gradually creep up over time.

I have spent the greater part of my adult life seesaw-
ing between 250 to 300 lb., being perpetually uncomfortable. This stopped four years ago, and I have been within
ten lb. of 220, either way, ever since. I have empowered myself with knowledge and positive actions. I am
choosing my own reality in the relativity of life—I have

changed my frame of reference. Whether it be a more positive parallel universe or whether it be a more positive probability is not the important thing—*the important thing is to choose.* You can choose, too. You must.

chapter fifteen

To swallow or to cut,
that is the question

I N EVERY SUNDAY PAPER you will find an advertisement for a product, a "fat burner" pill that will *melt
the pounds away* painlessly, without sacrifice. The
only way a pill is going to affect your weight is if it
suppresses your appetite, increases your metabolic rate,
or blocks the absorption of food. These drugs exist, but
I would only take them on the advisement of your physician. There are far too many unregulated products that
are of questionable efficacy, at best, to warrant your
attention or hard-earned money. The ads that promise
weight loss without changing your eating patterns are
the equivalent of those promising a free cruise or a way
to avoid paying taxes. If it sounds too good to be true,
then it most likely is not true.

Diet pills and supplements

When you read about vitamins and dietary supplements in throwaway flyers, it is hard to imagine living without them. Co-enzyme Q, chromium, CLA, assorted vitamins, Ningpo figwort root, foxglove root, *Rhizoma dioscoreae*, chondroitin sulfate, garlic: live longer, healthier lives; decrease risk of heart disease and cancer; live without pain. The ads typically promise something that seems essential or desirable and then they reference some form of "evidence" ranging from poignant first-person accounts to reports of "medical studies"—*studies have confirmed a significant loss of weight without changing lifestyle...*

The only valid study is one in which there is a control group that matches the study group demographically (age, sex, gender, race), and the ones administering the study don't know if they are administering the product being tested to the study group or the fake product to the control group; and the people receiving the pills don't know if they are receiving the actual product (study group), or the fake product (control group). The fake product looks just like the product being tested, and in the case of medications is often nothing more than a glycerin capsule or sugar pill. These studies are referred to as double-blind, randomized controlled trials (RCTs). They are expensive to do, for obvious reasons. I have reviewed available RCTs and reputable reviews of popular weight loss aids and have found none that document a *practically* significant, long-term weight loss. Studies quoted in the flyers and other advertisements are usually financed and administered by the companies marketing the products and often are of questionable, if not faulty, design.

There is also the question of safety. Recall the popular weight loss drug fen-phen, which was pulled from the market because of the associated risk of pulmonary hypertension. My feeling is that it takes five to ten years to *work out the kinks* of a new drug or invasive medical procedure. And don't think that just because supplements are OTC they are safe and do no harm. OTC drugs are less studied and less regulated than those medications that require a physician's prescription. The popular OTC stimulant ephedra was pulled from the shelves in 2004 after multiple reports of cardiac death related to the use of ephedra in labeled dosages.

Many vendors offer the initial purchase at sharply discounted prices, but soon a larger sum will be required, with prices ranging from ten to twenty dollars a month, or more. And if one supplement is good, then two must be better, and if two are better, then…*You would be amazed at the number of supplements some people take.* Perhaps you are one of these people. I suggest that you save yourself the expense of unnecessary, unhelpful dietary supplements. There may be a role for specific vitamin therapy but even the timeworn practice of a daily multivitamin has not been found to be particularly helpful. A recent medical study of 161,808 postmenopausal women, who took a multivitamin over an eight-year period, found no improvement in the risk of common cancers, cardiovascular disease or total mortality when compared to a matched group of women *who did not* take a multivitamin.[42]

Prescription diet pills

Appetite suppressants—act on the hypothalamus, which is the part of the brain involved in satiety. They are centrally acting stimulants, which means that they cause increased levels of epinephrine, dopamine, and norepinephrine in the brain. These chemicals are collectively known as catecholamines and they inhibit the brain's signal for hunger, thereby creating the feeling of satiety after a meal. The drugs available are sibutramine (Meridia), diethylpropion (Tenuate) and phentermine (Adipex-P, Fastin, Anoxine-AM). Side effects of the appetite suppressants can include increased heart rate, hypertension, and insomnia, because the net effect is similar to that of adrenaline or epinephrine, which is responsible for the *fight or flight response.*

Sibutramine is the only appetite suppressant approved for long-term use in the USA, being approved by the FDA in 1997. At least 29 RCTs have demonstrated efficacy. Three of the trials, totaling 929 subjects, showed an average weight loss of 9.46 lb. *more than the placebo control group* treated over a time course of at least one year.*[43]

Phentermine is approved for short-term use, 12 weeks or less. Although it has been around longer, there are fewer trials than those for sibutramine. One study of 108 subjects demonstrated a 5.8-pound weight loss *more than a placebo control group* treated over a course of nine months.†[44]

Rimonabant is an appetite suppressant available in Europe as Acomplia. It was going to be marketed in the USA as Zimulti; however, the FDA voted against its approval due to concerns of drug safety, as there was a suggested link to an increased risk of depression, anxiety, and suicidal thoughts.[44]

---

* In all of these studies, both groups lost weight due to the concomitant diet and exercise programs, but the treated groups lost 6–10 lb. more than the untreated group.

† See previous.

Fat blockers—inhibit a pancreatic enzyme, lipase, which is responsible for breaking down the fat in our meals so that it can be absorbed. The inhibition of lipase allows for a blockage of about 30 percent of ingested fat.

Orlistat (Xenical) is the only other prescription medication approved for long-term use in the USA. The primary action of the drug occurs within the intestine; only a small amount of the drug is systemically absorbed. Side effects include flatulence, oily or loose stools, and urgency. At least 28 RCTs have been completed that have demonstrated the efficacy of the drug as part of a program involving both diet and exercise. A total of 11 trials, comprising 602 subjects, of at least one-year duration demonstrated an average weight loss of 5.94 lb. *more than the control group.** [43]

In June of 2007, orlistat became available OTC as Alli, at half the prescription dose. A starter kit, with 90 pills (60 mg), can be purchased for fifty dollars. The studies of orlistat demonstrating weight loss that I reviewed were performed with the prescription dose of 120 mg, given three times a day.

The primary indication of the above drugs is for weight loss. Some physicians are also prescribing drugs that have a primary indication other than weight loss but which have a *side effect* of weight loss. These include antidepressants, anti-seizure drugs, and drugs used in the treatment of diabetes, sleep disorders, and attention deficit disorder.

Clearly, with the billions of dollars pumped into the diet industry yearly, there is active research under way in the development of better, safer weight loss prescription

---

*   See previous.

medications. Although the drugs used for the medical indication of weight loss have demonstrated statistically significant weight loss in RCTs, I would suggest that the differences are of questionable practical significance. Is an average weight loss of an additional six to ten pounds over the course of a year, which amounts to a daily energy deficit of 60–100 Calories per day, worth the cost and the inconvenience of taking a medication up to three times a day? More importantly, is it worth the potential risk of headache, hypertension and insomnia in the case of the appetite suppressants; or loose stools, urgency, and possible "leakage" in the case of a fat blocker?

With prescription drugs, some of the cost may be borne by insurance carriers and you might only have a co-pay of $5–20 a month. If not, monthly costs can run from $80 for full-strength orlistat to $180 for sibutramine, which are prices quoted from discount online suppliers. For long-term control, *ten pounds per year*, that amounts to an annual cost of $60 to $2,160, depending on the drug, and whether or not you have a low co-pay. Then you wonder: how long do I take the medication? Do I develop a tolerance? What happens when I stop? Do I gain my weight back? Let's say that you reach a target weight and quit your calorie-controlled diet and stop taking the prescription drug. Obviously, you will regain your weight, but this will have much more to do with the resumption of poor eating habits and a net positive energy balance rather than with the cessation of a drug that had a marginal effect in the first place.

The most significant benefit of a diet medication, prescription or otherwise, is the emotional and financial investments, which serve as handy reminders every time you lay down a Ben Franklin for a refill, swallow the pill, or pass a gut-cramping loose stool—*I am on a diet, I am on a diet, I am on a diet,* the little voice in your head whispers.

Would the diet pills be effective without a caloric restriction or, in other words, if you just took a few pills a day and ate whatever you wanted? I don't know. The only studies performed that I've found have dealt with groups with some caloric limitations. My hunch is that the answer is no.

Non-prescription diet supplements

There are so many different flavors of snake oil out there that it is difficult to find a place to start. The easiest thing to say would be *don't buy into this and don't take anything*; but advertising is powerful, and people, on the whole, are trusting and therefore vulnerable. Let me start with a summary of some summaries. These are reviews of quality studies of many types of diet supplements. Beyond that, I will address a few of the specific supplements that are commonly found, including a few that have actually demonstrated a subtle effect.

One comprehensive review of non-prescription dietary supplements from the April 2004 issue of the *American Journal of Clinical Nutrition* found no evidence beyond a reasonable doubt that any specific dietary supplement was effective for reducing body weight; none of the reviewed supplements were recommended for over-the-counter use.[45] The supplements reviewed included chitosan, chromium picolinate, *Ephedra sinica, Garcinia cambogia* (hydroxycitric acid), glucomannan, guar gum, β-hydroxy-β-methylbutyrate, plantago, psyllium, pyruvate, yerba maté and yohimbe. The only supplement which demonstrated an effect was ephedra, which had been taken off the market due to adverse side effects. The chromium picolinate had a small measurable reduction of weight as compared to placebo (0.08 to 0.2 kg/wk).

The Mayo Clinic website[46] has a summary of the weight loss supplements: bitter orange, chitosan, chromium, conjugated linoleic acid (CLA), country mallow (heartleaf), ephedra, green tea extract, guar gum, and hoodia. The site lists the claims of the various supplements, as well as the realities. Chromium is listed as relatively safe but unlikely to cause weight loss. CLA is listed as possibly decreasing body fat but not likely to reduce total body weight. The claim of green tea extract is increased metabolism and decreased appetite— the site suggests that there is limited evidence to support the claim. Hoodia is listed as an appetite suppressant but without conclusive evidence to support the claim.

Another review article from the December 2006 issue of the *Journal of the American Diet Association* was quite revealing.[47] The paper comprised an audit of 73 retail outlets that identified 402 products containing 4,053 separate ingredients. The mean number of ingredients per product was 9.9±8.96. A database search was performed for the ten most common ingredients, and only modest evidence was found in support of the effectiveness of green tea extract, chromium picolinate, and ephedra. The remaining seven—ginger root, guarana, hydroxycitric acid, white willow, Siberian ginseng, cayenne, and bitter orange—had inadequate or negative evidence.

A final source of review is the website consumer-search.com[44] that was updated in January of 2008. This site reviews all of the drugs already discussed and a few more. The salient point is a reference to a study of 15 reviewed supplements, of which five were identified as having potential promise with further study: pyruvate, DHEA, β-hydroxy-β-methylbutyrate, chitosan, and CLA. The same study concluded that the only supplement mix proven for weight loss was the ephedra + caffeine combination, which is a dangerous stimulant, no longer available. Further reference was made to a 2004 Harvard Medical School report stating that chitosan had no discernible effect on weight loss, and discouraged its use.

Many supplements are a potpourri of ingredients, not necessarily containing the supposedly therapeutic dose of any particular one. It is enough, I am afraid, to simply list an ingredient or supplement as being present and then the vendor can describe in detail how beneficial this or that ingredient is for you. There is often no oversight organization or regulating body, as is the case for prescription medications. Although there may be some voluntary oversight, the only mandated oversight that occurs is when something bad happens and people become ill, or die. This was the case with the prescription medication fen-phen and the non-prescription medication ephedrine.

Supplements with available studies for review

Conjugated linoleic acid (CLA)

CLA has been shown to increase lean body mass and decrease body fat mass in mice and rats[48,49]; therefore, it was immediately marketed as a weight loss drug, obtainable OTC, of course. *If it's good enough for rats…* Subsequent human studies have suggested that CLA may reduce the body fat mass at a therapeutic dose of 3.4 g per day. Long-term (1 yr) supplementation with CLA measurably reduces body fat mass and increases muscle mass in overweight adults, independent of any diet or exercise program[50]; however, there was no significant difference in body weight, because the loss of fat mass was balanced by the small gain in muscle mass. Additionally, there was no difference in the fat regain after the cessation of CLA. Another study also demonstrated that CLA did not prevent weight or fat mass regain in the obese population after cessation of the drug.[51]

In my estimation, the effect of therapeutic doses of CLA is questionable, with no significant change in body weight and a slight decrease in body fat mass in non-dieting, non-exercising adults. And this "effect" lasts only as long as the drug is being taken. At a minimum of $20 per month for a therapeutic dose, I do not feel it is worth the cost or inconvenience. $240 per year would be better spent on a health club membership, a nice set of dumbbells, or ten copies of this book to give to family and friends.

Green tea extract

The primary effect of green tea extract is via a DIT augmentation,[52] which we have discussed previously in some detail. The effect has been very helpful in rats[53]; alas, less so in humans.[54,55] In principle, there does seem to be some support for an increase in the metabolic rate, but this has not been adequately demonstrated in RCTs. As the effect is that of DIT, then it would make sense to ingest the extract before a meal, if you were of the mind to take it.

Although green tea extract is relatively cheap at $10 a month, my recommendation is still—*save your money.*

Hoodia

The active ingredient of the *Hoodia gordonii* succulent plant (cactus) is P57. The plant is considered to be an appetite suppressant that was brought to our attention by the San Bushmen of the Kalahari Desert, who used it to stave off hunger prior to long treks. It is also a protected species, threatened by extinction, which can only be harvested in the wild by individuals and companies with a proper license. Does it work? No double-blind clinical trials have been performed on humans; however, there has been some interesting work done on that rat population so fortunate as to be in the employ of man.

Rats who had P57 injected directly into their brains demonstrated a subsequent decrease in their 24 hr food intake by 40–60 percent. When the rat brains were sliced into tiny pieces and studied further, it was found that the ATP content in the hypothalamus was increased by 50–150 percent. In related studies, rats fed a low-calorie diet for several days (hungry rats) demonstrated a decrease in the ATP levels by 30–50 percent, but this decrease was blocked by injections of P57 into the rat brains.[56] It seems as though low levels of ATP in the hypothalamus are part of the mechanism of hunger and that when hoodia is injected into the brain, it causes an elevation in the levels of ATP, thereby creating satiety.

The bad news is that P57 is rapidly broken down by the liver. How much of this nearly extinct plant needs to be consumed prior to realizing any significant effect is unknown. When you eat hoodia, *it has to go through the liver first*. Apparently, the most effective mode of administration of hoodia is by direct injection into the hypothalamus at the base of the brain. Presumably, this

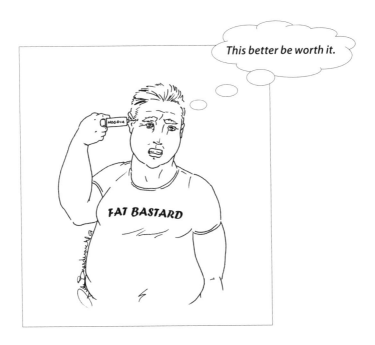

would be done with a large-gauge, six-inch needle that would punch through the sphenoid bone via a trans-nasal approach (through a nostril); not dissimilar to the movie *Total Recall* in which Arnold had to pull a tracking device out of his brain, also via a trans-nasal approach.

I think the most telling evidence against hoodia is that Pfizer originally owned the rights to the active ingredient P57 but released those rights in 2003 because it was too difficult and costly to isolate and synthesize P57.[57] Pfizer, as you may know, brought the world Viagra. If they cannot bring hoodia to fruition, who can? How likely do you think it is that small companies or organizations selling hoodia extract have solved this problem? How likely do you think it is that they even have significant concentrations of this nearly extinct, hard-to-cultivate plant from South Africa in their product? I think that the chance of significant weight loss from this suspect supplement is as likely as a rabbit's foot decreasing your time in a 10 k race.

Chromium

Chromium is a popular supplement. It has been thought to favorably alter body composition and enhance weight loss. Under conditions of controlled energy intake, chromium picolinate in the amount of 200 micrograms per day did not influence body weight or composition.[58] Additional studies looking at higher doses of chromium in conjunction with resistance training programs failed to demonstrate any enhancement of muscle strength or size, lean muscle mass, or body fat loss.[59,60]

Chromium pills are relatively cheap at less than ten bucks for a whole bunch. I suspect that the only benefit in caloric reduction is that obtained by the caloric cost of esophageal peristalsis from swallowing the pills and the metabolic energy required to warm to 98.6 degrees Fahrenheit the glass of cold water accompanying it.

7-Keto (metabolite of DHEA)

This steroidal hormone is now widely marketed after two studies of the products Lean System 7 and 7-Keto Naturalean demonstrated favorable results. The studies were eight-week random controlled trials that showed a 7 percent increase in the RMR. One of the studies documented a decrease in hip circumference of 3.78 cm in the study group versus 2.07 cm in the control group but no other significant differences in any other outcome variables. This represents a 0.7-inch difference in eight weeks. Unfortunately, the increase in metabolic rate did not translate into actual weight loss, but that wasn't mentioned in the abstract of the article or the lay publications.[44,61] I had to dig into the article to find that. At an approximate annual cost of $480, who would take a drug that costs that much and does not cause weight loss?

A final caveat is that these products are multi-ingredient supplements and Lean System 7 contains bitter orange, green tea extract, guarana and yerba maté, which are all stimulants, with the latter three containing caffeine. How much of the increase in the metabolic rate is due to the stimulant effect of this potpourri of ingredients other than 7-keto, which is promulgated as the "key agent"?

The use of herbal stimulants is not unique to a few isolated weight loss supplements; most are combinations of several OTC drugs containing stimulants which can have an additive effect. Bitter orange (*Citrus aurantium*) is a stimulant that increases the heart rate and constricts blood vessels. It is related to ephedra, which, as you know, was pulled off of the market. When bitter orange is combined with caffeine, the stimulant effect is accentuated. Now, mix in some other stimulants, like green tea extract and cocoa extract, and—POW! You might just stimulate yourself right into oblivion.

Dexatrim, Trimspa, CortiSlim, Lean System 7, Akavar 20/50, etc. are all such supplements containing multiple ingredients. To my knowledge, none have been subjected to double-blind, controlled studies in the scientific community, other than the two products with the "active" ingredient of 7-keto.

Marketing of OTC supplements

I think it is safe to say that we know, at least on a subconscious level, that just because we see something on TV, or read it in a magazine, does not mean it is true; especially if it sounds too good to be true. The unfortunate reality is that we tend to assign more credibility to these marketing efforts than they deserve. The problem is that we want to believe; we want an easier way without sacrifice or hard work. I think that it is basic human nature to be trusting, like a child, to believe in something that sounds nice and good. It is only after the punitive consequences of negative experiences that we learn to *not believe* in something that should be patently untrue to us in the first place.

Do not believe what you read in the advertisements for weight loss pills. Most of the time they are mere combinations of creative writing and lies, woven together in such a way so as to allow enough wiggle room to avoid legal liability. Let us take a closer look at just one full-page ad I recently tore from an insert of a Sunday paper publication.

A closer look at one supplement

"EAT ALL YOU WANT AND STILL LOSE WEIGHT? (And we couldn't say it in print if it wasn't true!)."

These are the largest letters, at the top of the advertisement. The entire background is in black; the typeface is compartmentalized in variable-sized boxes of different borders and colors. Nearly halfway down from the top of the page is a beautiful young lady with a seductive smile reclining on her side. This is the same woman that is on the

*website, except on the website she is wearing a bikini, and I
can see that in the paper advertisement she was Photoshop-
edited into a more modest one-piece suit, in observance of
the Sunday publication I am sure. I am to conclude that her
alluring figure is a direct result of the giant bottle of pills
that is positioned on the right side of the page, blocking a
view of shapely legs.*

"Introducing... ████████████ 'Fastest, Easiest Weight
Loss Ever'"

"STOP: READ THIS BEFORE YOU BUY ████████████"

"Fact: ████████████ causes excess fat to be pulled from
bulging parts of your body!"

"Fact: The secret is the formula...no need to count
calories."

"Fact: Clinical trial shows success...peer reviewed
clinical trial...23 out of 24 participants lost a significant
amount of weight."

"100 percent MONEY-BACK GUARANTEE!!"

"As with all our fine formulations, ████████████ is covered by our No-Nonsense Money-Back Guarantee. Our
guarantee contains no fine print or misleading terms.
Simply stated, if you use ████████████ and do not see...
just return the empty container within 30 days (we
would like you to use all of this fine formulation) for a
full, prompt refund."

I called their 1–800 number and asked the gentleman
who answered for the referenced articles. All he could tell
me were the names of two journals, *Psychopharmacology*
and *Journal of Human Nutrition and Dietetics.* He could
not give me dates, authors, or titles of the articles.

I then did an internet search on ████████████ and found
a posting from January 22, 2008, on the website, www
.sciencebasedmedicine.org, which described a similar

experience, except that the author pursued the organization over the course of two to three months, finally identifying the two articles. The titles of the two articles are listed as "Effects of caffeine, sleep loss, and stress on cognitive performance and mood during U.S. Navy SEAL training," and "Weight loss and delayed gastric emptying following a South American herbal preparation in overweight patients." The posting goes on to list the ingredients as yerba maté, guarana and damiana. According to the same posting, the patients in the study lost a few pounds initially, but then their weight stabilized over the next twelve months. The author had no further follow-up from the company.

The cost listed for the product was $39.99 for 60 capsules. The recommended dosing is one before each main meal. Assuming three main meals a day, sixty capsules would last twenty days. This leaves ten days to package and mail the empty container for a full refund (reportedly). This means taking the time and expense of repackaging the empty bottle, stopping by the post office during business hours, standing in line, and finally getting it sent off at a cost of around five dollars or so. How many people do you think will do this? Remember my earlier mention of the word "slippage?" Not only will most people not do this for a refund of forty dollars, but there is also the emotional aspect of admitting failure at something that supposedly works for everyone except you.

Retailers such as these do not make their money from repeat customers. They make their money from first-time buyers. Their quoted price is carefully calculated to be at the maximal amount that still allows significant slippage. There may be an occasional refund to a persistent consumer, but they would have to refund a significant percentage of their sold product before losing any money. These retailers are as ravens voraciously feeding on carrion at the side of the road. They will say or print anything to get you to buy their products. As far as I'm concerned, the only creatures that should eat their products are rats, since they're the only ones that the supplements seem to work for anyway.

The illogic of diet pills

Ultimately, it is a question of logic. It would be easy to spend a hundred dollars or more a month on dietary supplements, especially if two or more people in the household are taking them. What is the logic in taking supplements of little or no proven benefit and which may be a potential source of harm?

Consider the use of Xenical. At half the strength of the published studies, it would require a double dose of the OTC medication at a total cost of $100 a month. The medication blocks up to 30 percent of ingested fat. Using my 2,400-Calorie lifestyle as an example and 35 percent of those calories being from fat, this represents a blocking of 30 percent of 35 percent of 2,400 Calories, which equals 252 Calories a day. In a 160-pound person, applying the same parameters, this amounts to 150 Calories per day. In both cases, the same effect would be obtained from fifteen minutes of exercise, with the added benefit of an increased metabolic rate, the metabolism of visceral fat, improvement in cardiovascular and musculoskeletal health, and all the while saving $1,200 per year. On the other hand, 150 Calories a day does add up to 1.3 lb. a month. I suppose, if you feel the need to take *something* OTC, it would be this, *at this time*, as long as walking around with stomach cramps and smelling like a sewer doesn't bother you.

The diet medications that have the most impressive results are the appetite suppressants that we have reviewed, with a scientifically proven weight loss of ten pounds at one year, as opposed to six pounds at one year with prescription-strength orlistat. However, these medications are not OTC and require a physician's prescription. There is a new appetite suppressant, tesofensine, in the drug pipeline that may be about twice as effective as the current crop, but this is at least a few years from clinical use.

It is not that I am anti–easy weight loss, but I am anti-useless pills, some of which may cause harm. If a pill existed that was scientifically proven to safely allow an effortless and healthy way to a normal body mass index, I might be the first in line forking over some number of Benjamin Franklins, because that is how much it would most likely cost for a monthly supply.

Colonic irrigation

I recently saw another full-page ad on an inside page of a local newspaper, "Help Rid Your Body of Unhealthy Toxins." It made me angry because it was so blatantly misleading, yet I am sure these people will make thousands of dollars off of the ad.

"Reduce headaches, constipation; improve your immune system; look slimmer; and reduce excess weight … and on, and on …." It promises everything. The regular price of a healthy colon and all the attendant beneficial effects is only $49.00 plus $5.95 shipping; but, with the coupon in the paper you pay *only* $29.00 and the shipping is *free. Well, gee—what a deal—I'll get a couple.*

In the ad was a schematic of a terrible-looking colon, narrowed by schematic strictures and filled with schematic petrified excrement (before cleansing), and, of course, a schematically normal-caliber, clean colon *after a cleansing* with the product. With this product, the ad promises, you don't need to undergo the indignity of a high colonic, which requires gallons of water, and something akin to a garden hose inserted into a warm dark place.

I have done over ten thousand colonoscopies in my professional career, which means that I have cleansed over ten thousand colons. You don't need a high colonic or a colon cleansing to *clear out toxins*. A colon cleanser will not help you lose fat mass, it will not make "love handles" disappear. The only thing you will lose is money and a load of crap, which pretty much sums up the product itself. I am telling you the truth. Eat a healthy diet, high in fiber, as I am addressing in this book. Supplement your diet with a fiber powder, if necessary. If you still feel the compulsion to cleanse your colon, go to the local drugstore and buy a bottle of milk of magnesia for a few bucks and donate the money you've saved to the American Cancer Society.

Bariatric surgery

There are three types of surgical procedures for obesity: restrictive, malabsorptive, and a combination of the two. Restrictive procedures dramatically decrease the volume of the stomach, which limits the amount of food that can be swallowed at one sitting. Malabsorptive procedures bypass some portion of the small intestine, which decreases the amount of food (calories) absorbed.

Candidates for surgical treatment are patients with a BMI of greater than 35 who suffer from obesity-related illnesses like hypertension and diabetes; or, patients with a BMI of greater than 40. In the United States the most successful results have been obtained with the Roux-en-Y gastric bypass (RYGB), which is both restrictive and malabsorptive. With the RYGB a small gastric pouch (25 cc or 1 oz.) is created that is completely separated from the rest of the stomach—*restrictive*. Two to four feet downstream the small intestine is divided and hooked back up so that the gastric pouch bypasses those first few feet of small intestine, allowing for a decreased absorption of food—*malabsorptive*.

Less commonly performed is the biliopancreatic diversion with duodenal switch (BDDS). This is more of a pure malabsorptive procedure due to the fact that all but two to four feet of the small intestine is bypassed. Because of the severe limitation of absorption of nutrients, this procedure demonstrates not only the most impressive weight loss but also the highest complication rate and commonly requires future surgical revision.

Purely restrictive procedures that are gaining in popularity because of their less invasive nature are laparoscopic adjustable gastric banding (LAGB) and vertical banded gastroplasty (VBG). Thus far, the purely restrictive procedures have been shown to be 7–12 percent less effective than the RYGB, which is the gold standard for comparison in the United States.[62]

Results of bariatric surgery

A large study out of Sweden that was published in August of 2007 compared outcomes between two groups of obese patients: a control group that was managed medically, and a study group that underwent bariatric surgery. The study tracked outcomes for greater than ten years among the 4,047 obese subjects enrolled. Requirements for enrollment included an age between 37 and 60 years and a BMI > 34 for men and > 38 for women. In reading the study, I understood medical management to mean the medical management of the obesity-related illnesses, as well as dietary counseling. Whether or not the medically treated patients remained on a long-term diet is not specifically mentioned.

At the ten-year follow-up, in the control group (2,037 subjects), the weight remained stable at ±2 percent. In the surgically treated group (2,010 subjects), the weight loss was maximal at the two-year follow-up and after ten years the weight loss was 25 percent for the RYGB, 16 percent for the VBG, and 14 percent for the gastric banding. There was a significantly higher risk of mortality in the medically treated control group, with 129 deaths after ten years, as opposed to 101 deaths in the surgically treated group.[62]

The key point in regard to weight loss is that the average weight loss in the surgically treated group is some percentage of the excess weight. The majority of patients were still overweight, or less obese. The difference was enough to positively impact the long-term survival; but bariatric surgery rarely makes a thin person out of an obese one. For example, if I were morbidly obese, with a BMI of 40 (which I nearly was) at a weight of 319 lb., then a weight loss of 25 percent and 14 percent would have dropped me to the weight of 239 lb. (BMI 29) and 274 lb. (BMI 35), respectively—still uncomfortably overweight.

The key point in regard to the increased mortality in the medically treated group—no weight loss—is that *fat kills*. The most common causes of death from cardiovascular disease were heart attack, sudden cardiac death, and stroke. The most common cause of non-cardiac death was cancer. Please recall our discussions (*building blocks*) in an earlier chapter regarding the metabolic syndrome, insulin resistance and diabetes, the pro-inflammatory state, and the increased risk of cancer.

I have been in practice for fifteen years as a general surgeon. Just as I have never seen a thin post–bariatric surgery patient, I have also never seen an obese 100-year-old patient. I am not saying that they do not exist; rather, that I have never seen one personally. A recent paper out of Emory University looked at data from the Medicare population from ages 65 to 100 years of age and the researchers built a simulation model that demonstrated a convergence to normal weight of an elderly cohort.[63] What this means is that if you look at an elderly group of people, aged 80 to 90, they have, on average, a more normal body mass than a group aged 70 to 80. It seems that as *H. sapiens sapiens* ages, the obese people die off first—*there are really old people, and there are morbidly obese people; but there are no really old, morbidly obese people.*

Based on the available information, it is safe to say that bariatric surgery saves lives, but even a post–gastric bypass patient is going to require a lifestyle change if they wish to maintain significant weight loss, and doubly so if they ever desire to attain an appropriate BMI for their body type. Surgeons are interested in results; they will not operate on a patient who does not profess a commitment to the required lifestyle changes.

Bariatric centers therefore include dietary counseling and psychological evaluation as integral parts of the pre-operative process and post-operative care.

The malabsorptive procedures (RYGB and BDDS) are the only ones that may defeat a dysfunctional lifestyle, but they are also the ones with the most side effects and with the most risk of surgical complications, including mortality (dying). It is the malabsorptive component of the RYGB that results in its measurable, improved outcome when compared to the purely restrictive procedures. At the elemental level, the restrictive procedures are the equivalent of a "diet" in that they, at least initially, decrease the caloric intake by restricting the volume of food consumed.

Obesity surgery is a burgeoning industry, with 1.36 billion dollars of hospital costs being expended in 2004. This does not include the lifetime medical costs, which could range from $59,000–$75,000,[64] or the physician fees of $1,300–$2,000, which is what Medicare reimburses per patient. Of course, this seems cheap when compared to the estimated $100 billion health-care dollars spent annually on obesity and obesity-related illness.[65]

There are innovative companies making innovative products to perform bariatric surgery more innovatively. You see billboards on the highways and read about free consultations and bariatric surgery informational seminars given at local hospitals and clinics. Bariatric surgery is a solution, albeit an expensive one, but it does decrease the associated risks of obesity to a significant extent, as does the conventional successful diet.

My question is: if you have to be on a diet *after* bariatric surgery anyway, *why not go on a diet first?* I firmly believe that obesity and the recidivism of obesity are due to a lack of knowledge, an unenlightened state. We have been told all our lives that fat is bad and to eat multiple servings of high-carbohydrate-containing food groups per day. As far as I'm concerned, large segments of the general public have been ill-informed, in regard to nutrition, for the last fifty years. I appreciate the attraction of surgery, the immediacy, and the placement of trust in a highly trained professional to make you better—after all, I am a surgeon—but if there is an easier, safer way, shouldn't you take it?

Just as with diet pills, the patient makes an emotional and financial investment in the surgical solution, the difference being that this represents an investment to a much larger extent. In choosing the surgical solution, the patient has crossed a very significant bridge—he has literally chosen to lay his life on the line. I would suggest that there is much less of a need for the surgical solution in a population possessing awareness, in a population with the knowledge of the natural laws of our universe, and the courage and conviction to pursue a reality of their own choosing.

My belief is that if a patient (you) can cross that very same bridge without surgery; if you can be that committed to your health and well-being; if you can be inspired, motivated, compelled to approach your lifestyle modifications with the same level of intensity, as a matter of life or death, which it is, then success will be yours. Furthermore, if you can do this based on your own knowledge and empowerment, then your fulfillment will be increased tenfold and last all the days of your life.

And the answer is?

So to swallow or to cut?

That is for you to decide. You know what works and what doesn't. You know if it matters or if it doesn't, and if you think it's worth it, then that is your choice to make. You have been empowered to at least make an informed decision. Prescription diet medications and surgery are only crutches and very weak crutches at that. Even after spending all this time on our question, I am sorry to say that it is not the important question, because neither will carry you to that place where you want to be. At this point in time, both are as a flimsy bridge that is prone to failure. The crutches of pills and surgery are only marginally effective; and only then, if taken or performed against the backdrop of a change in lifestyle. Long-term weight loss will not occur by pills or surgery alone. It will occur only by you.

It is up to you to diverge from your present course. You live in a constant state of relativity in which much is possible. It is time for you to make the conscious choice to change your frame of reference.

Summation

Principles of the Diet Theory of Everything

1. *By thinking and acting positively, you increase the probability of a positive outcome.*
2. *It is much easier to consume 3,500 Calories than it is to lose it.*

3. *The natural tendency is to underestimate the daily caloric consumption of macronutrients.*
4. *If it's good enough for you, it's good enough for the rest of your family.*

Steps of the DTOE

1. *Be happy.*
2. *Calculate your appropriate daily caloric intake.*

$$\text{body weight in lb} \times \frac{11 \text{ Cal}}{\text{lb} \times \text{day}} = \text{Cal/day}$$

3. *Record your daily caloric intake,* RELIGIOUSLY!
4. *Monitor yourself,* BUT NOT TOO FREQUENTLY!

You will need to take ownership of your diet. You must write down your calories daily—it is energy, and only energy. Worry foremost about that and all the rest will follow, as night follows day. Remember these general guidelines, as previously explained.

Good carbohydrate	low glycemic index
Bad carbohydrate	high glycemic index
Good protein	low fat
Bad protein	high fat
Good fat	polyunsaturated, monounsaturated, and omega-3 (fish and nut oils)
Bad fat	saturated fats; hydrogenated fats, trans fats

Okay. Let's say a year has passed. You've lost several tens of pounds and achieved your target weight. You don't get short of breath going out to get the mail and when you pull your shirt off your torso ripples like a Spartan. *Yeah!!! Good for you!!!* Welcome to your new frame of reference. *Now what?*

Now nothing. What are you going to do? Are you going to stop eating the right things? Of course not. When you so carefully planned the lifestyle changes that fit with a calculated caloric need for an appropriate BMI those several months ago, the result was foreordained. The result is a product of the truth and universal law, and now, *nothing changes.*

The problem with a diet is that it is just a diet and, as such, something that is temporary. No one envisions being on a diet for the rest of their lives. According to *The American Heritage Dictionary,* the true definition of diet is *"the usual food and drink of a person or animal."* It does not mean a restriction in the caloric intake, which is what *diet* means to most people. You cannot go on a diet, reach a goal, go off the diet and expect to maintain your weight at the achieved target.

Unfortunately, most dieters who reach a goal are not committed to lifestyle change, due primarily to their unenlightened state. There is no resetting of the psychological set point, and previous dysfunctional dietary patters are reestablished.

How do I reset my psychological set point, you ask? By now, I would hope there would be no need to ask because the answer is before you in these pages—the awareness and knowledge of energy and the value of a calorie. Knowledge is power. Now you have the power. Congratulations and good luck.

chapter sixteen

Low-carbohydrate diet

LOW-FAT, high-carbohydrate, caloric restricted diets such as those historically promulgated by governmental institutions, *the Snickers bar diet equivalent,* work, but low-carbohydrate diets work better, and calorie/carbohydrate-controlled diets, *such as the DTOE,* work the best. Recently performed randomized controlled studies have addressed the specific question of low-carbohydrate versus low-fat diets in regard to the impact on weight loss and other health effects, and the evidence has come down on the side of the low-carbohydrate diets.

Although there may be a role for a more severe carbohydrate restriction in some cases, my goal is not to be a carbohydrate Nazi. Nor is my goal to discount the health benefit of whole foods that are carbohydrate based and that are good for you. Remember that our approach is that of balance and moderation. In the appendix I will

place a listing of healthy whole foods that should compose *a portion* of your diet.

I am not going to spend much time on specific low-
carbohydrate diets because I think it is a moot point at
this juncture. The fact is, by consuming an appropriate
number of calories, eating more protein rather than less,
and consuming lower glycemic index carbohydrates
rather than higher, you will, by default, be on a lower-
carbohydrate diet.

A review of two key studies

Gardner, et al.

"Comparison of the Atkins, Zone, Ornish and LEARN
diets for change in weight and related risk factors among
overweight premenopausal women: the A to Z weight
loss study: a randomized trial." Gardner CD, et al: *JAMA*,
March 2007, Vol. 297(9), pp. 969–977.

Number of subjects: 311

Description of the four diets that were compared

1. Atkins: very low in carbohydrates.
2. Zone: low in carbohydrates, with a ratio of
    40:30:30 of carbohydrates:protein:fat, respec-
    tively.
3. LEARN: lifestyle, exercise, attitudes, relation-
    ships, and nutrition: low in fat and high in car-
    bohydrates (50–60 percent), based on national
    guidelines—*not far from my Snickers diet.*
4. Ornish: very high in carbohydrates, vegetarian,
    emphasis on high complex carbohydrates, and
    less than 10 percent of energy intake from fat.

Before the study commenced, there was no difference in the percentage of energy from carbohydrate, fat, or protein. During the course of the study, there was a significant difference in carbohydrate content, as you would expect, in compliance with the respective diets. During the course of the study, there was no significant difference in regards to energy expenditure—no group exercised more than another.

Results

Mean 12-month weight loss

1. Atkins: 10.34 lb. with a range from 6.8–13.9 lb.
2. Zone: 3.52 lb. with a range from 0.9–6.2 lb.
3. LEARN: 4.84 lb. with a range from 1.8–6.6 lb.
4. Ornish: 5.7 lb. with a range from 2.9–8.4 lb.

Blood lipid measurements

- At all time points, the statistical findings for HDL-C (good cholesterol) and triglyceride concentrations favored the Atkins group.

Insulin, glucose, and blood pressure outcomes

- After 12 months there was no significant difference across the groups for either fasting insulin or fasting glucose concentrations.
- Parallel to the changes in weight, the decrease in the mean blood pressure levels was largest in the Atkins group at all time points of measurement.

Shai, et al.

"Weight loss with a low-carbohydrate, mediterranean, or low-fat diet." Shai I, et al: *New England Journal of Medicine*, July 17, 2008: Vol. 359(3), pp. 229–241.

Number of subjects: 322

Description of the three diets that were compared

1. Low-fat: restricted calorie, based on American Heart Association guidelines. Energy intake of 1,500 Calories for women and 1,800 Calories for men, with 30 percent from fat (10 percent from saturated fat) and a limit of 300 mg cholesterol per day. Low-fat grains, vegetables, legumes were encouraged.

2. Mediterranean: moderate fat (good fat), restricted calorie. Energy intake of 1,500 Calories for women and 1,800 Calories for men, with a goal of no more than 35 percent of calories from fat, the main sources of added fat being from olive oil and a handful of nuts.

3. Low-carbohydrate: non-restricted in caloric intake but restricted to 20 g per day for two-month induction phase and gradual increase thereafter to a maximum of 120 g per day. Vegetarian sources of fat and protein were encouraged, but participants were free to eat meat sources of protein at will.

After 24 months, the adherence rates were 90.4 percent in the low fat group, 85.3 percent in the Mediterranean-diet group, and 78 percent in the low-carbohydrate group. At the beginning of the study there was no difference in the composition of the diets of all the participants. The amount of physical activity increased significantly from baseline in all groups, with no significant differences in the amount of activity between the groups.

Results

Weight loss at 24 months overall

1. Low fat: 6.38 ± 9.24 lb.
2. Mediterranean: 9.68 ± 13.2 lb.
3. Low-carbohydrate: 10.34 ± 14.3 lb.

Blood lipid measurements/ inflammatory markers/blood sugar

- HDL-C (good cholesterol) increased in all groups, with the greatest increase in the low-carbohydrate group.
- The triglyceride levels decreased significantly in the low-carbohydrate group, 23.7 units of measure, as compared to the low-fat group, with only a decrease of 2.7 units of measure.
- The ratio of total cholesterol to HDL cholesterol, which is a ratio that your doctor checks annually, showed the most improvement in the low-carbohydrate group, with a relative decrease of 20 percent as opposed to a relative decrease of 12 percent in the low-fat group.
- The level of C-reactive protein, which as a marker of inflammation represents a negative, decreased significantly in only the Mediterranean group (21 percent) and the low-carbohydrate group (29 percent).
- In the participants with diabetes, the glycated hemoglobin level, which is a measure of blood sugar control (lower being good), was

significantly lowered in only the low-carbohydrate group.

The *Journal of the American Medical Association* (*JAMA*)
and the *New England Journal of Medicine* are two of the
most respected medical journals in the world. You will
not see these studies on paper inserts in the Sunday
paper or during commercial breaks on the television set,
which is unfortunate. These are not the only two studies
demonstrating these findings—they are two of the most
recent and well-done studies.

In both of these studies the most favorable outcomes were found in the low-carbohydrate groups, yet
the weight loss after one or two years was a modest
ten pounds on average. Most of the weight was lost in
the first six months, after which there was stabilization,
with a slight rebound.

A review of just one more study

Sacks, Bray, et al.

"Comparison of weight-loss diets with different composi-
tions of fat, protein, and carbohydrates." Sacks FM, Bray
GA, et al. *New England Journal of Medicine,* Feb. 26, 2009,
Vol. 360(9), pp. 859–873.

> Number of subjects: 811 (80 percent completion at
> two years)

Description of diets

> 1. Low-fat, average-protein (20 percent fat, 15 per-
>   cent protein, 65 percent carbohydrate)
> 2. Low-fat, high-protein (20 percent fat, 25 percent
>   protein, 55 percent carbohydrate)

3. High-fat, average-protein (40 percent fat, 15 percent protein, 45 percent carbohydrate)
4. High-fat, high-protein (40 percent fat, 25 percent
protein, 35 percent carbohydrate)

The *conclusions* of this article were "reduced-calorie
diets result in clinically meaningful weight loss *regardless of* which macronutrients they emphasize." This study
came out of Harvard and was sponsored by the NHLBI
and the National Institutes of Health—our old friends
of the Healthy Heart, Snickers bar diet equivalent. The
above ratios were suggested goals for the dieters, who
were periodically monitored over the course of two
years. The daily caloric intake was controlled *at the same
level* for all diet groups. Dietary guidance was given in
group sessions throughout the study period.

Results

Most of the weight loss occurred in the first six months.
Changes from baseline differed among the diet groups
by less than 0.5 kg of body weight and 0.5 cm of waist
circumference. At two years, 31–37 percent had lost at
least 5 percent of their initial body weight, 14–15 percent
had lost at least 10 percent of their initial weight, and
2–4 percent had lost 20 kg or more.

Risk factors

- All the diets decreased triglyceride levels simi-
larly, by 12–17 percent.
- Blood pressure decreased slightly (1–2 mm Hg),
with no significant differences between groups.

- The incidence of the metabolic syndrome at baseline was 32 percent of the participants, but ranged from 19–22 percent at the end of the study.

The data in this study was difficult for me to sort out, in contrast to the first two studies, because the diets weren't really divided into low- and high-carbohydrate, and in fact, there was no *conventional* low-carbohydrate diet, in the spirit with which we had been discussing, with the lowest carbohydrate restriction in the study being 35 percent. The other confounding factor in this study is the inherent difficulty in complying with a diet of such specific ratios over a time course of two years. I think that it was a poor study design, if one of the goals of the study was to disprove the efficacy of the low-carbohydrate diet that was suggested by the first two studies.

There are three key points that I would make with this study. Number one, none of the diets are low-carbohydrate *really,* and the one that comes closest is higher in fat than it is in protein. Number two, even a small amount of weight loss has a positive impact on obesity-related illness. And most importantly, number three: counting calories and controlling the daily caloric intake seem to have been the most important factor for weight loss in all diet groups. This third point is consistent with the first law of thermodynamics and the conservation of energy (*calories in equals calories out*) that I hope I have made clear throughout the text of this book. A final point I might make, if I were harboring a conspiracy theory, is that our government might be trying to make a point that isn't there, in regard to their exuberant and exclusive support of the low-fat, high-carb, Snickers bar-diet equivalent.

My conclusions that I have reached based on these and other studies

1. After only modest weight loss, there are significant improvements in health and a decrease in obesity-related illness (this is consistent with findings after bariatric surgery).
2. Calorie-restricted, low-fat diets do not work well and should not be promulgated by our government as the *only solution,* which has been the case for the past fifty years.
3. All fat is not bad for you, and it is an important part of the diet of *H. sapiens sapiens.*
4. The ideal diet for *H. sapiens sapiens* should limit carbohydrates to 20–30 percent (or less) of the total caloric intake during the weight loss phase, which is pretty much the opposite of the Heart *un*Healthy diet. As you approach your target weight, this restriction could be relaxed, with the appropriate foods, to more palatable levels.

Questions that I have based on these and other studies

1. How can a low-carbohydrate, higher-fat diet make me *less* fat?
2. Given that a high-carbohydrate diet increases insulin, which suppresses fat metabolism and encourages fat storage of excess carbohydrates, does that mean that insulin is bad?

3. How can I lose more than ten pounds in one to two years?

4. What is the effect of artificial sweeteners on insulin levels?

The first two of these questions are interrelated, and after consulting my 1986 edition of Guyton's textbook of physiology, whose pages haven't seen the light of day since shortly after 1986,[66] I have decided to approach these questions in a Euclidean fashion. I will review scientifically proven data in a list format, from which we will draw our conclusions. This is not new information or particularly earth-shattering information. It is merely oft-misinterpreted information.

Given—If given the choice of carbohydrate, fat or protein as energy substrates, the body prefers and will metabolize them in that order; carbohydrate first, fat second, and protein third. When given the choice of sugar or fat for energy utilization *at the same time,* the body will pick sugar first, always.

Given—All ingested carbohydrate that is not catabolized for energy is stored as glycogen for later use or synthesized into fat in the liver and adipose tissue.

- The glycogen energy stores are small, relative to the fat energy stores, and generally it doesn't take much glucose to replenish these stores—perhaps 50–200 Calories, unless the body is in a glycogen-depleted state such as with fasting or with a severely restrictive low-carbohydrate diet.

Given—All ingested protein that is not catabolized for energy or used for the processes of cellular structure and function is stored as fat in the liver and adipose tissue.

Given—All fat ingested that is not used in metabolic functions is stored as fat in the liver and adipose tissue.

Given—All carbohydrates cause elevations in insulin.

Given—The effects of insulin *as listed below:*

- increases the utilization of glucose by most of the body's tissues, which automatically decreases the utilization of fat.
- inhibits the action of hormone-sensitive lipase, which is the enzyme necessary to break the triglycerides into fatty acids, allowing the fat to be used as an energy substrate.
- promotes the conversion of ingested glucose, not required for cellular processes, into fat and transports it into the fat tissue for storage.
- promotes the transport of ingested fat, not required for cellular processes, into the fat cells for storage.
- promotes the conversion of ingested protein, not required for cellular processes, into fat and transports it into the fat tissue for storage.

Given—In the absence of insulin, fat is mobilized as the primary energy substrate.

- An example of this is in type 1 diabetes (juvenile onset), in which the metabolic defect is a lack of insulin production by the pancreas and the diabetic is thin from active fat metabolism. In contrast, the type 2 diabetic suffers from the metabolic defect of insulin resistance, the consequence being elevated levels of insulin, which promotes obesity due to excessive fat storage and the suppression of fat metabolism.

Conclusions that can be drawn from the above

1. Caloric intake that exceeds metabolic needs and glycogen replenishment, regardless of macronutrient source, is converted into fat. All excess ingested carbohydrate, protein and fat is turned into more fat.

2. From the standpoint of the first conclusion, the most important factor in weight loss is honoring the first law of thermodynamics: *energy in equals energy out,* or else there is an imbalance.

3. Since carbohydrates cause an elevation in blood insulin levels and insulin turns off fat metabolism and increases fat storage, then carbohydrates turn off fat metabolism and increase fat storage, especially when consumed in excess.

Carbohydrates = Insulin

Insulin = Fat

therefore,

Carbohydrates (in excess) = Fat

4. Insulin can be bad; *rather,* behavior (bad eating habits) that stimulates repeated surges of insulin is bad.

There are multiple problems with the calorie-restricted, low-fat, high-carbohydrate diet. The first problem is the lowering of the BMR that occurs without any specific measure to counteract it. When the body senses a caloric restriction from its baseline maintenance, its first instinct is to conserve energy by lowering the metabolic rate. If no effort is made to elevate the BMR with the previously discussed methods of aerobic and resistance training and DIT, then the decreased metabolic rate will significantly negate the caloric restriction. The second problem is the "turning off" of fat metabolism by carbohydrates. With the repeated ingestion throughout the day of carbohydrates and the concomitant elevation of insulin levels, glucose becomes the primary energy substrate and fat metabolism is suppressed. When glucose levels fall from the action of insulin moving glucose out of the bloodstream and into the cells, the appetite is stimulated, which triggers another rice cake snack and its subsequent insulin surge.

With the calorie-restricted, low-fat, high-carbohydrate diet, fat metabolism is diminished significantly and weight loss can only accompany significant, sustained caloric restrictions. Now, consider trying this diet in the morbidly obese diabetic patient, who already has elevated levels of glucose and insulin. Even if the carbohydrates are low glycemic index, they are still carbohydrates requiring insulin, which is secreted by the pancreas and/or exogenously administered. Is there any wonder at the high rate of recidivism of obesity?

This is the primary metabolic defect in the overweight and obese—the turning off of fat metabolism, which is a direct result of macronutrient ingestion. There is no genetic defect. There is no self-defeating biological set point. There is no magic pill that will make it better. There is only the cold hard truth—the reason *is sugar.*

With a low-carbohydrate diet, it doesn't much matter what else comes from what source, as long as the total caloric intake does not exceed the calculated need. Obviously, if you eat a lot of fat, you won't be eating much. For example, the energy in the pat of butter that you put on a baked potato is about as much as that in the baked potato—*oh, yeah, we don't eat those anymore, anyway.*

The more the carbohydrate restriction, the more the fat metabolism; this is why low-carbohydrate diets have an induction phase with a restriction of 20 grams per day, which can lead to dramatic initial results. Trying to eat less than 20 grams of carbohydrates a day in our society is virtually impossible, and, if you are not paying close attention to your total caloric intake at the same time, you are only a few slices of bread away from disaster.

I feel that an induction phase is reasonable for anyone, but more so in the morbidly obese individual, who is already at a significant disadvantage.* In the overweight or mildly obese individual, a more modest restriction of 60–120 grams a day in conjunction with the appropriate intake of the good macronutrients, as I have discussed, will be more palatable and easier to comply with.

The key is to keep it simple:

Count calories, eat lower-fat foods and low glycemic index carbohydrates, and look for foods with almost as much protein as carbohydrate.

You should realize that a protein entrée will offset the carbohydrate portions of your meal (fruits and vegetables)—remember—*balance.* As I have said several

---

* An induction phase should not be undertaken without the advisement of your health-care provider, especially if you are taking medications, or suffer from diabetes.

times, by doing this your carb-control becomes automatic. Do this, and it will take you where you need to be.

How can I lose more than ten pounds in one to two years?

To conserve and adapt—that is what our bodies do. If we decrease our caloric intake (especially with fasting), our bodies decrease the basal metabolic rate. If we train our muscles to perform a task, such as lifting weights or running a 10 k race, we will become stronger and faster over time. If we change our lifestyle and adopt an exercise program and change nothing, then our bodies will adapt over time and we will often plateau after an initial weight loss. Something needs to change going forward. We need to run longer or faster, or lift more weight or the same weight more often. Of course, if you are plateaued at your targeted BMI, then that is not such a bad thing, is it?

If you comply with your calculated daily energy balance, and by that I mean your diet in conjunction with exercise, your weight loss will begin to slow as you approach your targeted equilibrium point. This is the law of the universe: *energy cannot be created nor destroyed.* Your weight loss is inevitable.

We have already discussed maneuvers to increase the BMR and the effect of DIT. In the final section, the third and final pillar of the DTOE, we will address additional ways to accomplish a progressive weight loss.

What is the effect of artificial sweeteners on insulin levels?

This must be a good question because the answer is not readily available. Do insulin levels rise only in response to glucose, or do they also rise in response to artificial sweeteners? Although artificial sweeteners are not significant repositories of calories, if they do stimulate the release of insulin, then that would lead to a relative suppression of fat metabolism since that is what insulin does.

If this is the case, then drinking significant amounts of diet soda or ingesting other sources of artificial sweeteners, such as in tea or coffee, would certainly be detrimental to our goal of encouraging fat metabolism. One might assume that he or she can drink diet soda with impunity because of the absence of calories. After all, energy cannot be created out of nothing, right? True; but, if fat metabolism is suppressed, there may be a tendency for resting energy requirements to be met not by fat, but by the glycogen stores in the muscle and liver, which would then be replenished with the next meal.

Although I could find no human studies of the effect of various artificial sweeteners on blood insulin levels, there are several studies in the recent literature that suggest a link between soda and an increased risk of the metabolic syndrome and type 2 diabetes. It is interesting that both diet soda *and* regular soda have demonstrated this association.

One of the larger studies, published by the American Heart Association and involving thousands of subjects, clearly demonstrated the association of both diet and regular soda with the metabolic syndrome. In this study, the intake of one or more sodas a day was associated with a 50 percent higher incidence of the metabolic syndrome than in those who drank less than one soda a week. Additionally, there was also shown a 25–32 percent higher adjusted risk of the incidence of each of the components of the metabolic syndrome: obesity, increased waist circumference, impaired fasting glucose, higher blood pressure and high triglyceride levels.[67]

Another study of more than 2,000 subjects demonstrated an association of diet soda and significantly greater risks of two components of the metabolic syndrome, high waist circumference and elevated fasting glucose, as well as a greater risk of type 2 diabetes.[68] In this study, when the association of diet soda and the higher risk of type 2 diabetes was adjusted for baseline BMI or waist circumference (removing that variable as a possible cause) the associated increased risk of type 2 diabetes was not as strong, but still statistically significant. In other words, diet soda was associated with a higher risk of type 2 diabetes irrespective of weight.

An association of soda, whether diet or no, with the metabolic syndrome and type 2 diabetes does not prove causality; nonetheless, the association is concerning and would certainly suggest that, perhaps, we should limit our exposure to artificial sweeteners and refined sugar in general. There are a number of potential causes for the increased risk of the metabolic syndrome and type 2 diabetes found in the population of soda drinkers. For example, perhaps the soda drinkers have more of a propensity to crave sweets and eat more energy-dense foods, thereby suffering from weight gain and the attendant development of the metabolic syndrome.

What I wonder is, what if the increased risk of the metabolic syndrome and type 2 diabetes in drinkers of diet soda is because of its potential for the stimulation of insulin secretion? Is it possible that glucose tolerance and insulin resistance can develop from repeated surges of insulin from diet soda? Furthermore, if that is the case, then what is the long-term effect of repeated exposure to insulin from artificial sweeteners? Doesn't this mimic the obesogenic dietary pattern that is causative for glucose intolerance and the other attributes of the meta-bolic syndrome?

Boy, that's a lot of questions. Unfortunately, we don't have those answers yet. Historically, I have been of the mind that anything calorie-free goes. I never worried so much about drinking eight glasses of water a day because I figured that my eight cans of diet Coke sufficed. But now, I am questioning the assumption of the benig-nity of diet soda and artificial sweetener in general.

I know. I know. What is left? you ask. Water? Milk? Unsweetened coffee and tea? Orange juice that's half pulp? As I just stated, the definitive answer is not yet known, but the likely answer is, I'm afraid, yes to all of the above. I admit that I have been a voracious consumer of artificial sweeteners and diet sodas for as long as I can remember, including the past five years, during which I lost nearly a hundred pounds. When I started writing this book I remember looking for the answer, but all I found was a study from 1987 that demonstrated an increase in insulin secretion from the pancreatic islet cells in rats when they were exposed to concentrations of the artificial sweetener Acesulfame-K.[69] Because of this, and the above studies that became available for review more recently, I have markedly decreased my diet soda intake to less than one a day. Although I find this a little difficult, it is what I now believe, based on the evidence.

CITIUS, ALTIUS, FORTIUS

Faster, higher, stronger

chapter seventeen

Why exercise?

THIS LAST SECTION OF the Diet Theory of Everything addresses the third pillar of our trinity, that being exercise and the role of energy expenditure in our lives. This is not meant to be a comprehensive treatise on physical training for an elite athlete. This is what I consider the minimum. This is what has worked for Sue and me, and it will work for you. It may be that even the minimum is too much for you at this time. If that is the case, then start with half of the volume. Your fitness will improve rapidly and you will increase your volume in a relatively short period of time.

Too many people overlook the importance of exercise as part of a weight loss program and healthy lifestyle. Some might think that they get enough exercise cleaning their house or working at their job; perhaps they do if they have an eight-thousand-square-foot home or actively coach a wrestling program like our son

Jason. If that is not the case, then more is required of
Homo sapiens sedentarius. How much more? Five hours
a week for optimal results, of which three hours are
aerobic-based and two hours are involved in resistance
training.

A "side effect" of regular exercise is the endogenous
production of endorphins, which are neurotransmitters—chemicals that help nerve cells communicate.
They produce feelings of well-being, as well as providing *natural* pain relief. Exercise positively impacts
the neurotransmitters norepinephrine and serotonin,
which are thought to be factors in stress and depression. Regular exercise increases the serotonin levels in
the brain, allowing for a natural antidepressant effect.
I have been exercising regularly for four years and
am keenly aware of this effect of exercise. If I go more
than a few days without some form of exercise, I get
grouchy. It's kind of like I gnaw my way out of my baseline cocoon of kindness, grow horns and start acting like
Beelzebub.

Another "side effect" of regular exercise is an anti-
inflammatory effect, which offers protection against
all-cause mortality, primarily by protection against ath-
erosclerosis and insulin resistance. Regular exercise
stimulates the release of interleukin-6 (IL-6) by the muscle fibers. IL-6 is a powerful anti-inflammatory mediator
that induces the appearance of other anti-inflammatory
mediators, whose anti-inflammatory effects include the
promotion of lipid metabolism. IL-6 also inhibits the
pro-inflammatory cytokine tumor necrosis factor, which
plays a role in the development of insulin resistance.[70]
These anti-inflammatory effects of exercise are to the
metabolic syndrome what water is to fire.

Aerobic Exercise + Resistance Training = Balance

There is a general tendency to underestimate the importance of regular resistance training (weight lifting, isometrics, resistance bands). This is of specific value in women to offset the age-related development of osteoporosis. In fact, in regards to aging, I would go so far as to suggest that resistance training is as important, if not more important, than aerobic training. Each is of benefit, obviously, but in different ways. Let's say you choose one, exclusively, over the other. Consider my imaginary friends Joe Weightlifter and Jane Jogger for the purpose of illustration.

Joe Weightlifter lifted weights three times a week from high school until his death from coronary artery disease at age seventy-two. On the day he died, teeing off of the seventh hole at Apple Creek, he looked great. As he addressed the ball, his physique lent the impression of an old oak, thick and strong. His silk-and-cotton-blend knit shirt was stretched tight across wide, bulging shoulders. His good friend Reuben, who at eighty years of age yearned to be young and supple once more, marveled at the taut definition of Joe's ramrod-straight left arm during his backswing, brought into sharp relief by a bright morning sun. At the exact moment of impact, just after the impression of a well-struck shot flitted through Joe's mind, a five-millimeter plaque lifted up and occluded his left main coronary artery. Five millimeters is small, but so is the lumen of a coronary artery—Joe dropped to the turf like a sack of wet cement.

Although Joe lifted weights regularly, his cardiovascular system was rarely stressed beyond a few minutes at a time. He was a meat and potatoes man who preferred meat more, especially the red kind. When swimming, he sank like a stone due to his generous muscle mass wrapped around a robust skeletal structure. He thought that bike riding would make him impotent and that running was for wimps. He never considered the value of balancing his resistance training with aerobic training. The only time balance was important to Joe was during a set of squats with free weights.

Jane Jogger ran 15–20 miles a week from high school through middle age. By the time she reached her seventies Jane had decreased her mileage to a couple of miles three times a week. She maintained a trim figure throughout her entire life, the only change being her height. The inches melted away as her thoracic spine became increasingly more kyphotic from wedge compression fractures of the vertebral bodies, caused by osteoporosis. The natural age-associated loss of calcium from her bones, rather than being interrupted and reversed by musculoskeletal resistance training, was accentuated by its absence.

The overwhelming thought one had when seeing Jane Jogger running down the street was that she must have been running to a bell tower to swing from a rope. But beneath her hunched back, Jane's heart pounded away like a well-oiled metronome—lub dub, lub dub. Her preoperative cardiac clearances for bilateral knee and hip replacements were no problem whatsoever; and she will likely survive to be a 110-year-old, three-foot-tall woman, shaped like an upright comma, who wheels an aluminum walker with hand brakes up and down the sidewalk five days a week.

For Jane, the word "exercise" meant running, jogging, or walking—anything that increased her heart rate. She recognized the importance of stressing the cardiovascular system but failed to understand the importance of stressing the musculoskeletal system. To Jane, weight lifting was best left to men. She did not want to get all chunky and thick. The only time that balance was important to Jane was in bending over to tie her running shoes.

Balance. That is what we are about, as we have been all along. There are some fortunate few who are going to stand straight and tall and live to a ripe old age no matter what. I guess you would call that *good genes.* Take Winston Churchill, for instance. He smoked like a chimney, drank like a fish, lived to be ninety-one, and still managed to save the free world in his time here on earth. For those of us not so blessed, and since there is no way to really tell if we are so blessed, the safest thing is to assume that we aren't and institute a proper and sensible exercise program.

For those of you bemoaning a sluggish metabolism, this is your opportunity to be proactive and do something about it. As we have already discussed, there are three ways you can naturally boost your metabolism.

1. Eat every three hours to activate the DIT effect: try to eat at least half as much protein as low glycemic index carbohydrates on a gram-for-gram basis.
2. Aerobic training will increase the BMR by 10 percent.
3. Adding lean body mass (resistance training) increases the BMR 8–10 percent.

If you add all this up, you get an increase in your BMR well in excess of 20 percent.

Summary of benefits of exercise

1. Increase in basal metabolism. *Be thinner.*
2. Anti-depressant, feel-good effect. *Be happier.*
3. Anti-inflammatory effect that decreases risk of diabetes, heart disease and cancer. *Be healthier. Live longer.*
4. Assistance in maintenance of a healthy body mass. *Live stronger.*

Everybody knows that exercise is good for you, but not everybody knows why exercise is good for you. What I am telling you is the truth. I am not asking you to do this because it sounds good or seems right. I am asking you to do this because it is good. It is right. What you are learning is well researched, documented, and consistent with the truths and laws of our universe.

chapter eighteen

Energy nutrition

UNDERSTANDING THAT THE PRIMARY goal is that of weight loss, there are certain aspects of the metabolism of the three macronutrients that can be used to our advantage in attaining our goal. I think the easiest way to address this is to address the exercise metabolism of each of the macronutrients individually and then use that information to modify our exercise and nutritional patterns for maximal benefit.

Carbohydrate metabolism in exercise

We know from earlier discussions that the body prefers glucose above all else. We also know that one of the effects of insulin is the inhibition of the enzyme (lipase) that allows fat to be broken down into an energy substrate. It is not surprising, therefore, that the ingestion of a carbohydrate substrate will exert a two- to six-hour suppression of fat metabolism secondary to the rise in

insulin levels and the preference for the ingested glucose as the energy substrate. Eating a carbohydrate-
based meal or snack (bar) just before or shortly after the
start of exercise will produce less of a suppression of fat
metabolism than one eaten an hour before.[71]

The primary carbohydrate fuel source in mammalian
tissues is the complex polysaccharide glycogen, stored
in the liver and muscle tissue. During light to moderate levels of exercise, glycogen contributes little to the
energy requirements, which are primarily served by
fat. As the exercise intensity increases, however, so does
the glycogen metabolism, such that after two hours of
moderate- to high-intensity exercise the glycogen stores
are depleted and the energy requirements are then met
primarily by fat metabolism. With the depletion of the
glycogen stores there will follow a marked decrease in
athletic performance unless additional carbohydrates
are ingested.

The body's priority is to replenish glycogen stores;
it does this via ingestion of carbohydrate and protein
over the course of several hours. If a body is in a fasting
state post-exercise, then replenishment is accomplished
chiefly at the expense of lean muscle catabolism, since
only a small fraction (glycerol molecule) of the metabolic
products of fat can be converted into glucose. Conversely,
the ingestion of carbohydrate or protein or fat will have
a protein-sparing effect since the energy of the ingested
nutrients will provide glucose substrate for the brain
and allow a greater proportion of the body's glucose
sources to be diverted into glycogen replenishment. The
protein-sparing effect is more pronounced in the first
hour of recovery from exercise.

Opportunities for lifestyle modification

1. When you exercise at a low to moderate activity level, the primary source of energy is from fat metabolism.
2. When you exercise at a low to moderate activity level, there will be a minimal impact on the glycogen stores, which will be in a partially depleted state, most likely, due to a lower carbohydrate intake.
3. By timing exercise so that you eat a snack or a meal within an hour or two after finishing, you will realize a protein-sparing effect. This should not be hard to do, if you are eating every three to four hours.
4. If you are on a low glycemic index, low-carbohydrate diet, then it is not likely that your fat will be "turned off"; however, from the standpoint of fat metabolism, the *least favorable* time to exercise would be *after* a meal containing a larger proportion of carbohydrates.

Protein metabolism in exercise

When protein is catabolized, there are three possible pathways: the formation of a new protein, conversion to carbohydrate or fat, or further catabolism as an energy substrate. Although protein is not the preferred energy substrate, providing only 2–5 percent of baseline energy needs in a well-nourished individual, it is still a perfectly reasonable energy substrate. Unlike fat, protein can be a meaningful source of gluconeogenesis (glucose synthesis) and glycogen replenishment.

Because of the amount of protein turnover associated with heavy resistance training, the daily protein requirement will be higher, in the neighborhood of 1–1.5 grams per kilogram per day; but, if protein is already a significant proportion of the daily caloric intake, this then becomes a moot point. As with carbohydrate, the ingestion of protein in the post-exercise recovery period, sooner rather than later, will also have a protein-sparing effect, over and above that of the ingestion of carbohydrate alone.[72,73]

Opportunities for lifestyle modification

1. By exercising before breakfast in a fasting, glycogen-depleted state, you will maximize fat metabolism even at moderate levels of exertion, and the ingestion of a carbohydrate and protein (50:50 or so) breakfast within the first hour of recovery will exert a beneficial protein-sparing effect.
2. If it is difficult for you to exercise in a fasting state, then eat a higher-protein, low glycemic index–carbohydrate breakfast before exercising. This will not suppress fat metabolism as much as a high-carbohydrate meal, and there is the added benefit of DIT that further increases the metabolic cost of the exercise.

Fat metabolism in exercise

We know that fat provides up to 90 percent of the resting energy expenditure in a well-nourished individual, and that the body's fat stores contain enough energy for greater than 100 hours of high-intensity exercise. Much of the applicable fat metabolism has been addressed in

the carbohydrate section, but there are two further top-
ics that are of benefit to us.

We are interested in achieving maximal fat oxidation (metabolism). The maximal rate of fat oxidation has
been shown to be at exercise levels of intensity of about
60 percent in trained individuals and about 50 percent
in large samples of the general population. Endurance
training, with longer durations of exercise, will increase
fat metabolism further—in effect, you train your body to
become more efficient at metabolizing fat. As stated earlier, ingestion of carbohydrate before exercise will blunt
the fat metabolism by as much as 30 percent.[71]

Our final topic of fat metabolism in exercise is in
regard to excess post-exercise oxygen consumption
(EPOC). This refers to the elevation in metabolism following exercise, which lasts for several hours. Several years
ago, there was some initial excitement that the EPOC was
a major component of the daily energy expenditure and
that it could be utilized for control of body mass. There
are two key points regarding the EPOC. The first point is
that the exercise stimulus required to exert a significant
effect is out of reach of untrained individuals. The stimuli
involve either a submaximal exertion (70 percent effort)
for greater than 50 minutes or a supramaximal exertion
(105 percent effort) for greater than 6 minutes. The second point is that, even if these requirements are met, the
energy cost of the EPOC is only about 10 percent of the
net cost of the exercise itself.[74] In other words, it's a long
run for a short slide.

Opportunities for lifestyle modification

1. By using a heart rate monitor to keep your exertion level close to 50 percent, you can maximize

fat metabolism; and, as your level of fitness improves, you can increase your level accordingly.

2. By incorporating endurance training in the aerobic portion of your fitness program, you will metabolize more fat. Endurance training is not something that only highly trained athletes do—anyone can do it; all it takes is time. Riding a bike, power walking, jogging, swimming—any aerobic activity beyond 60 minutes qualifies. One or two endurance activities a week would be ample.

3. After reaching an appropriate BMI and level of fitness, you can vary your training by adding intervals of supramaximal exertion to realize the EPOC effect. This will make training more interesting and also will make you more competitive in local athletic events if you are so inclined.

Exercise-specific nutrition

In my unenlightened state, as a legend in my own mind, I had the impression that I was a competitive athlete, and therefore needed the proper nutrition for exercise. I bought protein powder supplements for my recovery from exercise, different powders to enhance my metabolism for higher-quality workouts prior to exercise, and I drank Gatorade during my workouts to avoid dehydration and to maintain intensity.

I didn't care much for my pre-exercise drink, but the post-exercise shake was top-notch: thick, creamy; made from 2 percent milk and a rich, chocolate powder. The only thing I didn't like about it was mixing the powder, which tended to glom up on the spoon and the sides of the glass. After breaking a couple of glasses with a metal spoon in my violent attempts to achieve a lump-free chocolate suspension, I was reduced to using a plastic baby spoon instead. Between my pre-exercise and post-exercise supplements, it seemed as though I was making as many trips to the health food stores as Sue was making to the cosmetic counters, and both were expensive.

Two thirds of the time my workout involved running, swimming, or biking at an exercise intensity of moderate to high, close to my lactate threshold, keeping with the spirit of *no pain, no gain.* My exercise time would average 40–90 minutes. I burned about 1,000–1,200 Calories per hour. During these periods of exercise I metabolized primarily glycogen for the reasons discussed above. The majority of my fat stores remained mostly untouched. Between the two and a half servings of Gatorade and the pre- and post-exercise supplements, I ingested over 500 Calories. My net energy expenditure was around 600 Calories. Since I metabolized mainly glycogen and since fat does not replenish glycogen, my fat stores were minimally impacted and continued to fulfill their baseline function of being the primary source of energy at rest. My glycogen was replenished over the next several hours from my dietary intake and the lactate and amino acids from the protein broken down during the course of exercise and subsequent muscle remodeling. The net effect was a minimal loss of fat mass and a mild increase in lean body mass.

With the goal of weight loss and decrease in body fat mass in mind, I had failed miserably. The moral of this story is to not get carried away with muscle milk and performance-enhancing drinks, powders, drops, or bars, unless you are Brett Favre or Lance Armstrong. Professional and elite athletes most likely do not need to lose weight and actually need the higher carbohydrate and protein intake due to their markedly elevated level of training.

There are many products that claim to increase the quality of your exercise session so that you can exercise at a higher intensity, which means you would be metabolizing mostly glycogen for the first 1–2 hours of exercise, if you go that long. If the primary goal is weight loss, is it logical to ingest *extra* calories to allow you to work out harder and suffer more, only to metabolize *mostly carbohydrate* at the expense of fat?

Save your money. There are benefits to eating shortly after exercise for the protein-sparing effect and glycogen replenishment, but *do not eat or drink more* than your calculated caloric intake for the day. *Everything counts.* I always make an attempt to eat something after exercising, either a meal or a snack, as a way of realizing the protein-sparing effect. My typical snack is a glass of skim milk, bar, low-carb wrap, or apple, although lately I've been experimenting with pickled pork hocks and turkey gizzards. As discussed earlier, there is some benefit to exercising within an hour after a meal for the enhanced DIT effect, *IF* that meal is low in carbohydrates so as to not blunt the fat metabolism.

Fifth Principle of the Diet Theory of Everything

The natural tendency is to overestimate the caloric expenditure of exercise.

This goes hand in hand with the second principle: It is much easier *to consume 3,500 Calories than it is to lose it.* Unfortunately, it's much easier to gain weight than it is to lose it.

chapter nineteen

What exercise?

ITH THE ASSUMPTION OF weight loss as the primary reason for exercising, the salient fact is that it doesn't have to be hard or unpleasant or boring. Unless you are training for peak performance, aerobic training should be relatively easy. As long as the primary purpose is weight loss and decrease in body fat mass, the effort level is only mild to moderate.

Aerobic training

The adage "No pain, no gain," is null in regards to aerobic exercise and decrease in body fat mass, because fat is the primary energy substrate for mild- to moderate-intensity exercise. As your exertion level increases beyond moderate levels of intensity, the muscle glycogen becomes the preferred energy substrate—at least, until it becomes depleted after about two hours. It is at this point of glycogen depletion that endurance athletes speak of "hitting the wall" or "bonking," which occurs when the body shifts to fatty acid metabolism. Unless further carbohydrates are ingested, the athlete will not be able to maintain the same level of intensity. To "burn fat" to a significant extent, therefore, you must either exercise longer than one to two hours at moderate to high intensity or exercise at a mild intensity however long you want. It's your choice. *I know what I'm going to do.*

How do I know what is mild to moderate?

The most available barometer to use is your heart rate. If you're too tired to check your heart rate, then you are exercising too hard. Another barometer is the perceived exertion level. This is a subjective scale, graded by how hard you feel you are exercising—a low to moderate intensity should feel that way. For instance, if you are jogging with a friend, you should be able to carry on a conversation of short sentences.

Monitoring your heart rate is the most accurate way to track your exertion level, and with a heart rate monitor it's also kind of fun. If you exercise at a health club or have a treadmill or equivalent, the machines may have contact handles with which to check your heart rate; alternatively, you can count your pulse at your neck for six seconds and then multiply that by ten.

To calculate your maximum heart rate, subtract your age from 220, which will give you an approximate idea. Generally, a mild to moderate level of intensity would be below a heart rate of 65 percent of the maximum (65 percent HR_{max}).

$$220 - age = \underline{\quad\quad} (HR_{max})$$

This is your maximum heart rate.

$$HR_{max} \times 0.65 = \underline{\quad\quad}$$

Write it down.

This is the heart rate that you should stay under in order to burn all that nasty fat.

For myself, the calculation is

$$220 - 45 = 175 \ HR_{max}$$

$$175 \times 0.65 = 114$$

I know this well because I perform the bulk of my aerobic training at this level and it is not hard. I can do this for over an hour. I quit only when Sue needs my assistance with the gardens in the summertime, stained glass caning in the wintertime and sewing projects all year long.

What kind of aerobic exercise should I do?

I prefer to swim, bike, or run because of my interest in triathlons; but aerobic exercise can be anything that maintains a consistently elevated heart rate for more than a few minutes. If you are a morbidly obese person who can't tolerate any of the above, then I would simply start with walking for twenty minutes no matter how far you get. It will get better from there. I promise.

Types of aerobic exercise

- Walking
- Jogging
- StairMaster
- Elliptical trainer
- Bike riding
- Swimming
- Jumping rope

In our aerobic exercising we must not forget the importance of *gravity.* Gravity is good. In performing the work
of exercise, it is helpful to review the actual formula for
work that you may recall from school: work equals force
times distance.

$$W = F \times D$$

Where

> W is work
> F is force
> D is distance

While we all know what *distance* is, let's examine *force*
more closely, from the standpoint of Newton's theory of
universal gravitation, in consideration of your gravitational mass.

$$F = G \ \frac{m_1 \times m_2}{r^2}$$

Where
> G = gravitational constant = 6.67×10^{-11} newtons
> m_1 = mass of a body (you)
> m_2 = mass of a body (earth) = 6×10^{24} kg
> r = distance between two point masses,
>   in this case = radius of earth = 6,360 km

What the above formula tells us is that our gravitational
mass (weight) is directly proportionate to the weight of
the earth. Obviously, if the earth were twice as big, we
would weigh twice as much. This is why astronauts on
the moon could take twenty-foot steps. Moreover, from
the above, it is also apparent that someone with a larger
gravitational mass will perform more work for a given

distance than someone with a smaller gravitational mass. When I go walking with my lovely wife, for instance, I am performing nearly twice the work she is, which means that I am expending nearly twice the calories and should get twice as much dessert—*a high-protein, low-carb dessert, of course.*

What you will also notice is that there is no factor of time in $F \times D$, where F is considered roughly equivalent to mass, which means that it doesn't matter if you cover two miles in twelve minutes or half an hour. The caloric cost is the same.

You can use gravity to your advantage in aerobic training. Gravity is partly responsible for the work you do and the calories you burn. If you take gravity out of the equation, such as with bike riding, you will likely burn fewer calories per a given time at a given heart rate. With the goal of weight loss in mind, therefore, use weight-bearing aerobic exercises to increase the caloric cost.

If there is a desire to accentuate the caloric expenditure of walking, try wearing ankle weights. Walking is a relatively low-impact exercise, and with the extra weight carried *below the knee* (ankle weight) the added force will not be transmitted through the knee joint. This is in contrast to a Special Forces soldier training with a rucksack of rocks on his back, which I wouldn't recommend, unless you are fond of orthopedic surgery.

Fifth Step of the Diet Theory of Everything:
Perform three hours of mild to moderate aerobic activity a week.

This sounds like a lot if you are doing nothing currently. It is not that much. Do you spend time watching TV or news programs, listening to broadcast radio or reading?

These are all activities that can be performed simultaneously with an aerobic activity performed at a mild to moderate level of intensity. I'm a nut for political cable news programs. I don't know why, because I just get frustrated; consequently, I don't watch them nearly as much anymore—but I used to. Most evenings, when I used to watch them more often, Sue would find me in the spare bedroom, sweating profusely while pedaling away on my recumbent bike.

During these fat-burning marathons I'd frequently violate my self-imposed moderate-exertion barrier because of the talking heads going at it on the screen in front of me. Invariably the conversation would evolve into a viewpoint antithetical to my political views and before long, my legs would be pumping like pistons, as though I were the reincarnation of Lance Armstrong barreling down the Champs-Élysées. I'd find myself sucking down ragged gasps of sweat-steamed air, and just before coming to my senses, I'd realize that I was screaming… *I really can't say—Sue made me edit it out of the book!*

I have no difficulty in finding time for aerobic activity as long as I tie it to TV, which is particularly helpful in the wintertime. I feel better about it, as though I'm accomplishing something productive—*exercising that is, not watching TV.* If I watch TV and I'm not exercising, then I feel like that's a waste of time. Today, I rarely watch cable news unless I am exercising. I read books on my elliptical trainer and upright stationary bike. It is amazing how time flies in the pursuit of fat oxidation.

It doesn't particularly matter if you do one hour every other day or one hour for three consecutive days. The most important factor is a three-hour weekly volume. If meaningful weight loss is a goal, optimal results will be obtained with exercise sessions of at least sixty minutes or with a caloric expenditure in excess of 400 Calories. This means that it is better to do three one-hour sessions rather than six thirty-minute ones. You will be pleased to know that, as your fitness improves, and you plateau at an appropriate BMI, you will be able to maintain your level of fitness with lesser volume. At this level of fitness, or any level, really, an occasional slow week due to a vacation or work is easily absorbed.

Resistance training

Use it or lose it. If you never had it, get it. You can—it is never too late. Proof of this is found in the results of a ten-week study of one hundred nursing home residents with an average age of 87 years, enrolled in a resistance training program. This was a study to demonstrate the utility of weight lifting for seniors. The average increase in muscle strength was 113 percent.[75]

If you stop resistance training, there will be a reversal of gains—this is called detraining. After two weeks there are significant losses in muscular strength and aerobic capacity as well, if that is also a component of your training. After four months of cessation, all gains are lost, as though they never were.

With resistance training, not only do the muscles get bigger and stronger, but the tissues that attach the muscles to the bone (connective tissue) also thicken and increase in strength. Because of stronger connective tissues—ligaments and tendons—the joints are strengthened and become more resistant to injury and the ravages of time. Additionally, bone mineral density, as a measure of osteoporosis, correlates positively with muscular strength—this just gets better and better.

Quick, someone give me a dumbbell. One, two three four, Two, two three four…

Misconceptions

1. *Weightlifting will slow me down and negatively impact my flexibility.*

   Truth   Flexibility will improve. There is no decrease in range of motion across joints or decrease in limb speed.

2. *Weight lifting will make a woman bulky.*

   Truth   Weightlifting increases tone and shapeliness, unless bulk is the goal, in which case the woman must eat two chickens a day, and spend six hours a week in the gym with a bunch of hairy, sweaty, grunting men with body odor—*Sue might like this, but not most women, I suspect.*

3. *Weightlifting requires a lot of time with lots of sets for good results.*

   Truth   For the goals of muscular strength, with its attendant benefits and weight loss, only one to two hours a week is needed. I will outline a specific program of two sets of exercises, each with 10–12 repetitions.

4. *Exercise equipment is expensive.*

   Truth   It is, at least for quality circuit training equipment and a heavy-duty treadmill; the cost could easily exceed two thousand dollars. On the other hand, all you really need is a good set of dumbbells or resistance bands, some core body aids such as a Pilates ball, and nice weather; or a fitness club membership. Basements all over the world are filled with barely used exercise equipment, tucked into corners and lined up against walls. Sharply discounted, high-quality, slightly used equipment is yours for the taking. All you have to do is evaluate the used equipment at fitness stores or research local newspapers ads, and buy from the *unenlightened.*

In the appendix I have outlined a resistance training program that will take one hour to complete. A large part of it was shown to me by Jessie's former boyfriend, Tom, of our previous Casablanca acquaintance. Tom was shown this routine by his personal trainer and good friend, Jerry. Tom and Jerry do about nine hours of resistance training a week, so I imagine they know what they're talking about.

I have slightly modified Tom and Jerry's routine so I wouldn't kill myself, or anyone else who I chose to share it with. This series of exercises is what I have come to call the *Phalanx*, in reference to the ancient Greek military formation of armored men. Historically, the phalanx consisted of a mass of soldiers in several ranks (rows); the soldiers in the second rank projected their spears over the heads of their compatriots in the first rank, who linked their shields together, collectively projecting a wall of armor. Just as King Leonidas and his force of 300 held back the Persian hordes at the battle of Thermopylae with the phalanx, so will we hold back the ravages of time and obesity and osteoporosis with our modern-day *Phalanx*.

I taught the Phalanx to three people. Within six weeks, two of those people, who were women, received compliments on their arms. The third person, Commander Kluge, went off to war in the Middle East, and when he returned he had a torn rotator cuff and looked about the same as when he left. I know that many women are self-conscious about their upper arms. The Phalanx and the DTOE bring a quick resolution to this self-imposed self-consciousness.

I showed Sue the Phalanx a few weeks after I had been doing it. This was the year of her braces, so every two weeks she had to go to her orthodontist for a two-hundred-dollar adjustment. One day, after six weeks of the Phalanx and six hundred dollars of adjustments, she was in the doctor's office with the dental hygienist, who asked, "What on heaven's earth is going on with your arms?"

Puzzled, Sue replied, "Ah, what do you mean?"

"Well…they're so toned. I want arms like that."

Sue explained how I had shown her these exercises, and she found herself doing the Phalanx, sans weights, until the orthodontist walked in, wondering, I'm sure, *what the…*

Around that time at work one day in the endoscopy room, a couple of the staff, Kurt (the commander) and Gina, coaxed me over to the YMCA to show them the Phalanx. I ran them through the paces and got them all qualified on the regimen. Not six weeks later Gina was running on the treadmill when a lady came up to her and exclaimed, "My God. What have you been doing with your arms? I want arms like that."

Sixth Step of the Diet Theory of Everything:
Perform two hours of resistance training weekly.

This includes the Phalanx, core muscles, and a few leg exercises.

These are outlined in the appendix.

The complete regimen will take approximately one hour.

What I am describing is what Sue and I have been doing the past three years. It is very similar to the position statement on physical fitness published by the American College of Sports Medicine. It is interesting and gratifying to see that what I arrived at independently, based on my research and personal experience, is quite in line with the position statement of the American College of Sports Medicine (www.acsm.org).

chapter twenty

Motivation

WHY EXERCISE? WHY DIET? To what end? There are the specific reasons that I have just listed: increased metabolism, antidepression, anti-inflammation, and weight loss. The final common pathway of these and other positive actions, positive outcomes and optimism has something to do with living a longer, healthier, happier life. For some people, the goal is more finite—*I want to look drop-dead gorgeous for my best friend's wedding*; or, *by golly, my ecotour to Tibet leaves in two weeks, I'd better get in shape.*

For others, the motivation might be a specific event—a turning point in their life after which nothing is quite the same. It might be the loss of a close friend, a diagnosis of cancer, a heart attack—or some other close encounter with mortality that precipitates a change in outlook, an appreciation for every day, an appreciation for the privilege that our life is. Such was the case with me.

It began one dark and stormy night in January of 2001 with chest pain—pain that I had been dealing with for days, blaming it on muscular soreness from the labors of moving our daughter to the University of Wisconsin at Whitewater. I sat at our kitchen table, slumped over and sweating. Sue felt my forehead and her hand felt good, smooth and cool against my skin.

"It feels like you're burning up, and you're soaking wet. Let's take your temperature."

By the time I got to the bathroom I knew something was seriously wrong. I couldn't seem to get enough air. I took my temperature. It was 102 degrees. One hour later I was lying in the emergency room of my own hospital listening to the soft murmur of voices from behind the desk. The emergency room physician, Martin, was a good friend of mine. Through the opening in the curtain of my cubicle I could see a view box with a chest x-ray hanging on it. It looked like the chest x-ray of an eighty-year-old man in congestive heart failure because the heart shadow filled up the whole chest and the lungs were white instead of black.

Oxygen from the nasal cannula calmed my breathing. What could be wrong? A list of diagnoses sifted through my mind, with a few rising to the top. It was a quiet night. When Martin came in to talk to me I said, "That's my chest x-ray, isn't it?"

"Yes, I'm afraid it is."

I recalled all the nights of sweating spells and low-grade temps that I had been experiencing in the months leading up to Jessie's move. "I'm in some sort of leukemic crisis, or maybe lymphoma?"

"It's likely. I'm so sorry, but you're in pretty tough shape. I'm bringing the CT crew in to scan your chest."

Martin took my hand, squeezed it. "You might want to call Sue."

I had driven myself in because it was late and, well, I didn't think it'd be anything that serious. My nurse brought me a phone and left the room, closing the curtain completely behind her.

"Hi, honey," was all I could manage to say.

"Shaun, are you okay?"

"It doesn't look too good, babe."

I could hear her sudden intake of breath. I felt her love, and then, her fear. I was suddenly in a cocoon of her emotion, alone, in my curtained room. "I think I have lymphoma," I whispered.

"What does that mean?" But she knew. The anguish and love in her voice were more than I could bear. The cell phone felt warm in my hand and I couldn't say anything. "I'll be right there." And then she was gone. I was alone again, and I felt strangely light. The chest pain eased and I could breathe without feeling starved of air.

The time between my brief conversation with Sue and her arrival was most peculiar. I have never felt it before, and have not experienced it since. Although the voices around me were quiet, I still could hear them clearly inside my head. As I lay there dying, or so I thought, the ceiling tile seemed close and I noticed the symmetrical pattern of its perforations, as though they were right before my eyes, rather than ten feet above me. For the first time in my life it was like there wasn't a thought in my head, but I was present—I heard, I saw, I smelled, I felt. In the next room I could hear two women softly crying. I imagined that someone had died.

The CT scan showed that I had a large pericardial effusion, meaning that there was fluid around my heart,

trapped inside the pericardium, which is a sac that surrounds the heart. My heart couldn't beat effectively
because of the fluid, and the pericardium was inflamed,
which was causing the chest pain. My eventual diagnosis was chronic relapsing pericarditis. I underwent
emergency surgery the morning after my presentation
to the emergency room. Unfortunately, it did not solve
the problem and over the next few months I experienced the same debilitating symptoms every month, like
clockwork, lasting a week at a time. After three months
of failed medical management I was scheduled for surgery at an academic center with a world-renowned chest
surgeon, who happened to have performed the world's
largest series of radical pericardiectomies. He lived six
hours away from me, by car.

May 1st of 2001 was my date with the professor, or, at
least his fellow; perhaps a resident, maybe. For all I knew,
he could have let a file of medical students step up to the
table, one at a time, to take turns tearing away strips of
my inflamed pericardium. Whoever did it did a wonderful job. This I know, because I'm still here.

My post-operative course was relatively unevent-
ful, other than overdosing on morphine. I was using a
patient-controlled anesthesia pump, which means that
if I felt pain I pushed this little red button on the end of
a cable. The button had a very easy action with barely
any resistance and if there hadn't been a tiny electronic
beep that sounded, I wouldn't have been sure I actually
pushed it. So, I pushed a button that felt like it wasn't
there, a muted electronic beep sounded like a solitary
chirp of a lone bird perched on the IV pole next to the
bed, and two milligrams of morphine sulfate squirted
into a dorsal branch of my cephalic vein.

My difficulty arose when I had this bright idea that if I dosed myself in anticipation of pain, *before I felt pain,* then I wouldn't have to feel any pain. Given the level of my obesity and the volume of distribution of morphine in lean muscle mass, and a medical student calculating my morphine dose based on my weight, and a resident who complied with the attending's order to *give him what he needs* when said attending found me howling in pain on my first post-operative day, my electronically heralded squirts of morphine apparently added up to quite a bit.

I figured I was overdosing because I wasn't breathing as much as I felt I should, my head was spinning, and I was nauseated. Swimming in an opiate-induced languor, I was thinking: *I don't have cancer, thank God. But now, after all this, I'm going to die of asphyxiation from over-dosing on morphine, compounded by my obstructive sleep apnea from being fat.*

My nurse didn't seem to think I was overdosing; con-sequently, she wasn't as concerned as I was. She changed her mind, however, just before her shift ended and right after sitting me up in a chair. The phone rang. I answered. Out of nowhere, a wave of nausea welled up and all I did was open my mouth. I didn't think to keep my mouth pointing in any one direction, like down at the bed or towards the emesis basin on my nightstand. No, instead, I looked frantically about the room, at the phone, at the ceiling, and at the nurse. I think that I was more sur-prised than anyone else by the fountain of vomit shooting from my mouth in rhythmic contractions that slammed against my fresh sternotomy wound like a sledgeham-mer. The pain was incredible, despite the overdose. It felt as though there was fire flaming out of my chest with each pulse of vomit. After my brief but dramatic display of projectile emesis, I wiped my mouth with a handful of Kleenex and said to the nurse, "I told you I was over-dosed on morphine."

During my five-day stay at the academic center, there were torrential rains and tornado warnings. My wife and youngest son, who were with me, had to leave their hotel to seek safety elsewhere. They came to the hospital, where they found all the patients out in the hallways, except me. Later, they told me how they had looked for me, and then found me alone in my room, next to a big plate glass window. I don't know if I was the last one to be moved or if my nurse just never got around to it.

I now believe that my inflammatory pericarditis was due, at least in part, to the pro-inflammatory state of my obesity; but at the time, in my unenlightened state, the cold breath of mortality was enough of a motivation for me to lose weight, again. This time, after a three-year process of enlightenment, it took hold.

With good health as my primary motivator, I began swimming at the local YMCA. I used to think that I was an excellent swimmer for the simple reason that I could hold my breath underwater for two minutes. I was wrong. I was a lousy swimmer. I knew this when a lady with blue hair sticking out from underneath a swim cap passed me doing the breaststroke in the next lane. Everyone swam faster than me. It took me forty strokes to cross a twenty-five-meter pool and halfway across I'd have to routinely wave off the lifeguard running towards me with a body hook. I looked like a broken human propeller—there was nothing smooth about my stroke. It took as much energy for me to swim twenty-five meters as it takes Michael Phelps to swim a mile.

Determined to overcome my disability, I joined the masters swim class at the YMCA. Thankfully, there was a patient, kind soul there who was genuinely interested in my becoming a better swimmer. Thanks, Mike. I never became a great swimmer, but I stopped embarrassing myself, I like to think.

Nemesis

Another powerful motivator for exercise is to find a nemesis. I found mine in my sheep-farming anesthesiologist friend, Brutus, who was also a swimmer, only a real one. Brutus swam competitively in high school. He also wrestled, was a track star, and fenced. Brutus did everything. One day at the pool when swimming next to him, I noticed that I had managed to swim 1,500 yards without my sternotomy incision hurting. So I said, "How about a hundred-meter race after Easter, Brutus?"

Brutus stiffened. I could see the not so fine hairs on the back of his neck and on the back of his back in general rise up in a primordial Neanderthal-like fashion. Little did I know what fury I had just unleashed—I swallowed hard. He growled, "you're on," and as he turned away I heard him mutter under his breath, "I'm going to kick your ass."

During the next four months, leading up to Easter, Brutus swam like he was training for the Olympics. He joined the masters swim class as well, and started brownnosing Mike, like a high school student infatuated with a pretty teacher, so that it was hard for us other students to get any quality attention. The Monday after Easter, in the quiet of an afternoon, with no one watching, Brutus beat me by three fourths of a pool length.

The following Christmas, during a party, he suggested that we enter a sprint-distance triathlon at the
end of July. I remember him saying that it would be *just
for fun*. I told him that it sounded like a great idea, thinking that maybe I had a chance, *like maybe one in a billion*,
of actually beating him, but I knew it would be a great
motivator for exercise.

All that winter Brutus pestered me with questions
about how my training was going, what I was doing, how
much I was swimming. I was purposefully vague. I didn't
share the results of my research on aerobic base training or running efficiency. Every now and again he would
shoot me a time; *I swam five hundred yards in eight minutes today,* he'd say. I never reciprocated.

In the spring Brutus suggested we go for a bike
ride at his place, on his route along the lake. He had a
Schwinn aluminum-frame 10-speed bike, left over from
high school. I was driving a carbon-frame Trek road bike
that was the same model that Lance had won the Tour de
France with, a few years earlier. We took off, and within
minutes the farm was far behind, and so was Brutus. I
slowed down, like when I go bike riding with Sue. Brutus
pulled up next to me a few minutes later.

"Man, I think it's my bike," he said.

"Here, let's switch. I'll put my seat down and you put
yours up."

"No, no, that's okay," said Brutus.

"Oh, don't be silly. I want you to see how a real bike
handles."

Brutus pedaled off on my carbon frame. It took me
a few minutes to get used to his archaic shifters of an
early-eighties vintage, and he pulled a few blocks ahead.
A few minutes later I passed Brutus, thinking that he

was taking his time, savoring the responsiveness and lightness of my OCLV carbon frame with all the top-end trimmings. Brutus wasn't savoring the top-end trimmings. I slowed down, again, to my biking-with-the-wife pace until he caught up, out of air and muttering, "Damn, damn, damn, it's *not* the bike."

It took him two weeks to recover from my victory, because I don't think it ever occurred to him that I might be better at something. Brutus bought a triathlon-specific bike, trained until he got saddle sores, and then trained some more. On the day of our first sprint triathlon, he beat me by a full eight minutes, and his bike split was just a whisker over mine. Brutus is now a competitive age-grouper at the half-ironman distance.

This July will be my fifth sprint triathlon. This one event, which consists of one hour and some fraction of another, keeps me exercising all year long. The training is a combination of swim, bike, run, which is a wonderful variety. I add resistance training, and each year, as I get older, I get stronger and faster.

Body image as a motivator

Another common motivator is body image. How do I look? In our current culture there is an emphasis on thinness—an ectomorphic body habitus. Western civilization's concept of beauty was established several hundred years ago by Greek and Roman artists. The typical body habitus was that of a mesomorph—well-muscled and long-legged, with a head of thick hair. Michelangelo's *David* was the epitome of male beauty at that time and still is today.

This was recently brought to life in the movie *300*, which depicted a battle between 300 Spartans and

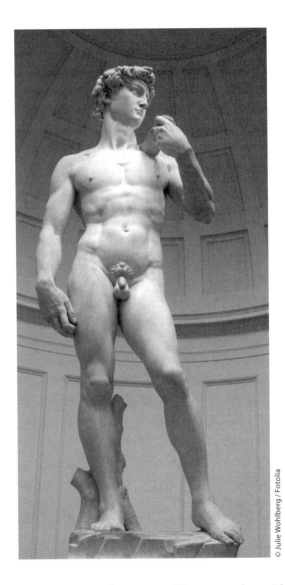

© Julie Wohlberg / Fotolia

thousands of Persian forces at Thermopylae. Although outnumbered, the Spartans managed to defend the passage between narrow cliffs until they were eventually surrounded and killed.

I have never seen as many heavily muscled physiques in one place before as in that movie. It was like watching the *Iliad* come to life. I doubt that there was one male in that theater who didn't want to look like a Spartan, me included. I knew that if I had a six-pack and shoulders like that nobody would ever kick sand in my face again. Skinny? Thin? Hells bells, I want to be a David. I want to look like I just crawled out of the mind of Michelangelo. I want to ripple like a Spartan.

Citius, altius, fortius; the third, and final, pillar is *perfectus* (finished). You know what you need to know.

Now, go forth, you, the Spartan within, and manifest yourself.

POST-ENLIGHTENMENT

Employ your time in improving yourself by other people's writings, so that you shall gain easily what others have labored hard for.

Socrates

chapter twenty-one

Singularity

E BOTH HAVE COME a long way. You, in reading my book, and I, in writing it. To the old adage "You are what you eat" I would add another: "You are what you read." As you have read these pages, know that I have learned along with you, and that is due solely to the intellect of men and women who have put their thoughts into words.

We began our journey of enlightenment with emotional health because it is so important to address any pathology at that level, which may be a factor in being overweight or obese. If there is emotional ill-health and if it is part of the cause, if it is not resolved, then the goal of long-term weight loss becomes more elusive.

I have shared a way out of the darkness by daring to contemplate the mysteries of our universe and the physicality of what we are. I do not understand it, whether it be God or science, or a combination thereof; but whatever it be, I know this: I know it to be indeterminate. This means that the course of our lives, meandering through the space-time continuum of our ephemeral existence, is charted by none other than us.

⧚

The first step of the DTOE, *be happy*, is fulfilled by adhering to the first principle:

By thinking and acting positively you increase the probability of positive outcomes.

The first principle is fulfilled by adhering to the tenets of our Western civilization and the golden rule, or simply— to do good things.

It is very likely that you will be able to find your way out of the darkness of emotional harm by yourself; but, if not, please seek the support that you require.

⧚

The middle portion of your journey to enlightenment dealt with the conservation of energy and how it must be honored in regard to achieving an appropriate energy balance. The energy balance will initially be negative (losing weight), with an eventual progression to zero as your body mass plateaus at an appropriate BMI.

This second pillar encompassed these principles:

It is much easier to consume 3,500 Calories than it is to lose it.

> The natural tendency is to underestimate the daily caloric consumption of macronutrients.

and

> If it's good enough for you, it's good enough for the rest of your family.

The first two principles are honored in complying with the following steps of the DTOE:

> Calculate your daily caloric intake.

> Record your daily caloric intake religiously.

and

> Monitor yourself, but not too frequently.

In choosing the right types of macronutrients with the correct proportions at the right times, you will begin to lose weight, which is mostly space, as we now know.

> Count calories, eat lower-fat foods and low glycemic index carbohydrates, and look for foods that have almost as much protein as carbohydrates.

Do these things and weight loss is as inevitable as the changing phases of the moon.

♯

The third portion of your journey, the third pillar, was the briefest. And if you were to surmise that is because it is the least important, I would not protest too much. Nonetheless, exercise or energy expenditure over and above that of the RMR is an important part of reaching your goal. It does not have to be hard or painful if the primary purpose is that of fat metabolism, since the exercise is performed at a low to moderate exertion level.

The third pillar encompasses the fifth and final principle:

The natural tendency is to overestimate the caloric expenditure of exercise.

As efficient as our bodies are, it does not take as much energy as you would think to perform a physical activity, relative to the energy we consume. The energy burned in a thirty-minute walk will not negate a piece of rum cake. On the other hand, with a larger body mass, more energy is consumed with physical activity; so a thirty-minute walk would negate a piece of rum cake if you were eight feet tall. I earlier used an example of exercising with my wife. If the two of us go on a slow run at, say, low to moderate exertion, at the end of thirty minutes I will have burned 600 Calories to Sue's 300–400 Calories (I can't say exactly because that is a big secret). This means that I get three fourths of the piece of rum cake.

Aerobic exercise and resistance training are of equal importance and require a small fraction of your time over the course of the week. There are timing factors and macronutrient choices that can be applied as opportunities for lifestyle changes to maximize fat metabolism.

In the appendices that follow I will include the one-hour resistance training regimen that helped me to be like David. However, resistance training regimens can be found anywhere, and it does not matter so much what you do as it does that you actually do it.

Finally all the building blocks are in place. Singularity is near. You know what you need to know. You hold the stone of empowerment in your hand—it is almost time for you to leave. I could stop writing now, but I would like to carry you along a bit farther on your journey into the positive reality that you have chosen—a reality, or a probability, that was fulfilled the very instant you opened the cover of this book and began to read. I understand that the DTOE was not short. I understand that the DTOE was not easy. And, unless you were keeping notes as you read through the book, you are probably thinking, *what the hell do I do now?*

Do this. Acquire the things on this list.

1. The courage to change (free)
2. Calorie counter ($8.00)
3. Small tablet and pen ($1.00)
4. Scale ($12.00)
5. *The South Beach Diet Cookbook* or other lower-carbohydrate, good-fat recipe book ($17.61)
6. Heart rate monitor ($50.00)
7. Set of dumbbells ($100–300) or
8. Set of resistance bands ($25.00)
9. Ankle weights ($25.00)

Cost: $338.61

Cost of a body that crawled out of the mind of Michelangelo: priceless.

Refinement of dietary recommendations

Everything that I have written pertaining to the science of weight loss is factual and referenced. It is not made up or a matter of opinion; however, what follows is. Based on what I have learned and on my personal experience, what I am going to now suggest is my *opinion* on the best approach to weight loss.

Based on my research regarding the hormonal actions of insulin, I am of the mind that a lower-carbohydrate diet facilitates fat metabolism and thereby weight loss. Clearly, there are health-care professionals who will tell you that low-fat and caloric control are key and that low-carbohydrate diets don't have additional benefit. Well, all I have to say about that is, *this is my book, not theirs.*

For subjects with a BMI of < 38

You have less than one hundred pounds to lose. You most likely are at least in the initial stages of the metabolic syndrome, if not further along. I have devoted an entire chapter to the low-carbohydrate diet, and I would suggest reading it again. As I have stated numerous times, by controlling the calories in, restricting carbohydrates to low glycemic index ones, and making an effort to pick foods with at least as much protein as carbohydrate, you will, by default, be on a reasonably low-carbohydrate diet.

In that spirit, you do not need to specifically count carbohydrates unless you want to. If you do, I would anticipate a daily intake of around 100–200 grams, which would be around 30 percent of your daily caloric requirement. I do not feel that an induction phase is necessary, although, if you are so inclined, I am not opposed. The problem with an induction phase is that it is very restrictive and requires a great deal of planning and effort to comply with unless you are a hermit, never leave the house, and have lean meats and vegetables delivered to your door. Weight loss results with an induction phase can be dramatic, especially when you comply with the calculated caloric requirement.

If you do decide on an induction phase of < 20 grams of carbohydrates a day, I would not get too carried away by continuing it much more than a few weeks. Also, realize that you will be in a chronically depleted glycogen state and physical activity at moderate to high levels of effort may be difficult.

For subjects with a BMI of > 38

You have nearly a hundred pounds or more to lose. You are most likely suffering from the metabolic syndrome, if not already diabetic, and may have significant underlying heart disease—*this risk increases with age*. This means that you should enlist the aid of your physician for co-management. You need to have your blood tests checked. You need to know your cardiac status and if you will tolerate physical activity of a moderate level without injuring yourself. You may need closer monitoring of your blood sugars and changes in insulin dosing if you are diabetic.

I am sorry to say that your fat metabolism is virtually nonexistent. This can only be reactivated by taking carbohydrates out of the equation. In this case, an induction phase will be helpful for two weeks, alternating with a regular low-carbohydrate week (100–200 grams), or some alternating pattern such that you don't go bonkers and turn into a carbo-Nazi. Once your BMI is south of 38 you may forgo the induction phase forever.

DO NOT drastically alter your diet (induction phase) without guidance from your physician. Doing so could result in dangerous metabolic disturbances, and that would make me feel bad. Your lifestyle change will need to be a collaborative effort between you and your doctor or a licensed dietician.

Final dietary comments

There is a little-known factoid about starvation that most people don't know, probably because few have actually been in a starving situation. And, I don't mean that period of time between breakfast and supper. The curious reality is that when you are starving (beyond the first few days) you really aren't all that hungry. However, if you have a six-week supply of rice cakes, rationed out at three per day, you will be constantly ravenous. Carbohydrates make you hungry; protein and fat do not—protein and fat cause satiety. On a low-carbohydrate diet, therefore, you will be less hungry than on the equivalent low fat, high-carbohydrate diet similar to the Snickers bar diet or the diet that the government, at least historically, would have had you eat.

In the appendix that follows, I will list snacks and foods that I have on hand *if I just gotta eat*. I will also include a short list of healthy whole foods. Lastly, I will summarize all of the lifestyle modifications and opportunities that I have touched upon throughout the book.

Time management comments

A common complaint with unenlightened dieters, as well as some freshly enlightened ones, is time—*but, but, but, I don't have the time for that*—*that* being the time required for food preparation and exercise. I don't know what more I can say, other than *Where there is a will, there is a way.*

I think that television is a chief culprit. It certainly was for me, until I gave it up three years ago. I went from watching two to four hours of broadcast TV a day to four hours of broadcast TV a week (while exercising). In between those two extremes was eighteen months of no broadcast TV. Although my abstinence from TV was not intended, it did have unintended consequences. I experienced an incredible burst of productivity, including the time to research and write this book in the time left over from a demanding surgical practice in which I was on call 50 percent of the time. I have read shelves of wonderful books that would not have received a second glance in my unenlightened days. I have completed a multitude of complex and extravagant landscaping projects and many more menial gardening chores under the capable instructions of my wife, the gardener.

The precipitous happening, which triggered such a dramatic change in my life, nearly ended in tragedy and was addressed in elaborate detail in my Christmas letter of 2006. If not for this, I would most definitely be in a completely different universe—one in which I weigh 350 lb. and am sitting in front of a 60-inch plasma TV watching a twenty-four-hour cable news channel and eating sour-cream-and-Ranch-flavored Doritos from a 20-serving bag.

MERRY CHRISTMAS 2006

After a few minutes of sitting on a rubber mat in my basement, in the lotus position, staring at a potted plant, deep in Tran meditative thought, awaiting enlightenment, I realized that my knees were killing me and that the only enlightenment I'd ever achieve would most likely be pharmacologically induced. Howsoever, I did, after a few recitations of some silly mantra—I think it was "rum cake"—decide to pen a final Christmas letter for the faithful. I say 'faithful' in reference to those who have already inquired about my letter this year and also those who have expressed appreciation for them in the past.

I say 'final' because it could be. None of us can know God's plan, and this past August as I nearly fell to my death it didn't occur to me at the time that gee, last December was my last Christmas letter, and if I had known that, I suspect it would have been different. Imagine the poignancy of each day if you thought it was going to be your last. Imagine the energy it would take to sustain that day after day. Although it may sound noble and virtuous to say that I'm going to live every day like my last, or write a letter like it might be my last, it is not realistic, unless I really knew it was my last. So I can only make transient approaches towards the ideal. If tomorrow (Monday) were my last, I would still wake my wife with a kiss like I do every day, but, after that, much would be different. Maybe this Christmas season, like the eve of Christmas Eve or the day after Christmas, or some other time quiet, you could call someone you haven't talked to in a while who you care about and talk to them like it was your last day, but just don't tell them that or they'll think you're crazy.

I've sometimes thought that there must be a master plan and that I, as everyone, have a specific role to play— destiny, a special purpose, whatever. A few times after a significant event, where I knew that I made a difference— like this one time when I found an early prostate cancer in a forty-year-old during an army physical, knowing that he never would have been checked otherwise—I wondered if I had fulfilled my special purpose and was ready to go back to Mother Earth or Father Sky. I think it is safe to say that I am not yet done, given the events of 14 August 2006.

I found myself on the roof of my fortress of solitude over a matter of principle. It has been my experience that in matters of principle it is the principled one who suffers the most, for the simple reason that when you do something "for the principle" usually it's because there is no other good reason. The "principle" often costs more or has some other intangible expense, perhaps relating to convenience or enjoyable pastimes—like watching Packer games or the fair and balanced Fox News.

The matter of principle in this case related to a poor experience with an unnamed satellite television network. I never did like all the channels. I found them confusing, and I could never seem to find what I was looking for anyway. Consequently, I didn't watch much programmed TV other than the news channels and, of course, Packer games. I did record HD movies on the provider's DVR and would watch these most often but then, one day, the DVR broke. After about 3–4 hours of invested time via automated phone trees, tech support and email, followed by a week of anxious waiting, I eventually got another DVR, which was exactly like the one I had sent back that was three years old. Within two weeks I was having exactly the same problem. After about 20–30 minutes of automated phone time, I finally found myself talking to a live customer agent for the still unnamed network. I explained my problem and asked, "Surely in the past three years there must be a new and improved DVR that has come along?"

"Oh, of course there is," said the female voice, "but that's a $200 upgrade."

"But I paid $400 for this one."

"It's still an upgrade."

"Well, I don't want satellite television anymore."

"Sorry, there's nothing I can do."

"I quit. I don't watch all that much TV anyway and have been paying over sixty dollars a month for a service I'm not utilizing."

"You'll have to send the equipment back," she threatened.

"Okay."

"Even the LBF on top of the roof," she said ominously.

"What…how do I take that off?"

"All you need is a Phillips screwdriver…three screws."

"But I thought I bought all that stuff. Like I said, I paid $400 for the DVR."

"That was a lease."

Somewhere around a month later, on a hot August afternoon, I found myself on the westerly slope of the roof of my house.

I had my right leg wrapped around the southerly strut of the satellite dish support and was twisted, like the infinity sign, so that I could see the undersurface of the thing that looks like a microphone that the lady said I had to send back with the receivers if I really wanted to quit the satellite network because of lousy service. In my left hand I held a poor copy of three different dish configurations, none of which looked like mine, which as I recollect was the SUPER-DOOPER SATELLITE 3000 GT or some such thing that was twice as expensive as the standard version. In my right hand was the Phillips screwdriver that the lady said was all I'd need.

The paper said something about a housing and three screws, and all I could find were two, which were recessed into the housing such that I couldn't really see if the Phillips was mated with the head of the screw. It took me about ten minutes and several F'enheimers to get those out. My lovely wife, who had insisted that I wait until she returned from Wal-Mart before starting my roof work, monitored the situation from the second-level bedroom balcony.

Obviously, there was yet a third screw, since I could twist the housing this-a-way and that-a-way but not lift it off. I tapped it and gave it a few good tugs just to make sure and then after stretching a bit further, and a few more *foot-pounds of torque on my anterior cruciate ligament, I discovered the wily, again recessed, screw in a most inconvenient location. I made sure that Sue knew how hard I was working for us by grunting a few more expletives as I wiped my sweat-drenched brow with the back of my hand. The third screw came loose, slipped out of my fingers, and rolled twelve feet down the 8:12 slope into the rain gutter as I finally ripped the housing free.*

Unfortunately, in waving the housing triumphantly for Sue to see, I only made the hornets, in the nest on the inside of the housing, angrier. I have been petrified of bees ever since one stung me on my neck right over the Adam's apple when I was four, but I had that coming as I was for some reason whipping a small bees' nest in a juniper bush with a chain I made from beer and pop can tops (the kind you had to be careful about swallowing long ago). The difference this time was that these weren't friendly honeybees; au contraire, *these were two-inch yellow jackets from South America that sounded like buzz saws, probably this far north because of global warming.*

Naturally I screamed and threw the housing (to hell with the refund) as far as I could. My sweaty right leg slipped from the strut and I thought I saw Dakota (my dearly departed black lab) waiting for me at the bottom of the hill. The only thing that kept me from rolling off the roof and plunging three stories past our lovely walk-out basement onto the two-story slope littered with jagged, dead tree trunks and boulders was a wet, soft body and the coefficient of static friction of scorching, black asphalt shingles on a hot summer day.

Now you have an inkling of why I've been referring to our home as the fortress of solitude—we have no TV, our only newspaper is the local bi-weekly which is bereft of national news, radio is so "yesterday," and our Internet connection is abysmal and shuts down if we try to download a wallet-sized photo. This forces Sue and me to spend

much time together and, instead of the background din
of cable news programs and football, there is instead
the sound of constant Christmas music, ninety percent
being Sarah McLachlin and the Trans-Siberian Orchestra.
Perhaps that is why, after four months, solitude remains
at 4081 Shoreside Drive, other than our lovely family and
friends whose occasional visits we enjoy so very much.

Sue and I are truly blessed to have each other and our
beautiful family. Sometimes I have to pinch myself just to
make sure that this vision of loveliness is with me still, after
all these years. We would like to wish all a Merry Christmas,
God's blessings, and a healthy and happy New Year.

I am not anti-TV; in fact, I enjoy watching it very much
and look forward to the movie rental that we receive in
the mail 1.5 times a week. I know that it would be easy
for me to slip back into the habit of watching broadcast
TV more frequently, so I make the choice to not watch it
at all unless I'm exercising or if a Packer game is on, or
both. I know that there is probably a parallel universe
inhabited by a hyper-obese Shaun Melarvie watching TV
24/7 while eating Snickers and cookie-dough blizzards;
but that is his universe, not mine.

As I sit down to write this last chapter, it is Wednesday. I am off every other Wednesday and it is my weekly
weigh-in. This morning I weighed 219 lb., which is a BMI
of 27, which puts me only at "overweight" with a moderate health risk. I know that this is inaccurate because I
have slain the Goliath of obesity with the stone of empowerment. I have unleashed the Spartan within.

Sue and I were in Omaha last week visiting our two-
year-old granddaughter, Evie. The first morning of our
visit we took her to Graybar Park, four blocks away. Sue
pushed an empty stroller while Evie jogged with me at

her side. She ran with a wide-based, shuffling gait, like her father; that is to say, like a muscle-bound wrestler with chronic low-back pain. She insisted on being in front, taking comfort in my advancing shadow to her left. It was a beautiful spring day, with a sky so blue that it hurt her eyes to look at it. I could not help but wonder what exponential number of photons was striking the earth around us, and I looked forward to the day when she would be old enough for me to explain shadows to her.

At the park I pushed her on the adult swing as I swung next to her on an adjacent one. By chance, we were in rhythm. I marveled at our two radically different gravitational masses falling to the earth at the same accelerated velocity of 32 feet per second per second. We relished the rush of air and weightlessness of free fall on the downswing and the increasing inertial weight on the upswing until reaching the zenith of our arc, at which point we were momentarily suspended in air before being pulled back by the gravitational force-vector of the center of the earth.

I shouted out to Sue the seemingly remarkable observation that Evie and I were swinging at the same speed even though I was so much heavier. I thought of Galileo dropping objects of different mass from the parapet of the Leaning Tower of Pisa 425 years earlier. How it must have felt to be the first man to make the same observation, only blessed with the awareness to realize its significance.

⚌

Two years has passed. I am still working on the last chapter. I had thought it well finished previously; but then something happened that I'd rather not get into, and another something also happened, which I would like to share with you. This, however, requires a brief back-story.

Since we have been living in our house on the side of a hill, an entire clan of robins has built a veritable robin-condominium project in the rafters of our upper-level deck every spring. I remember the first year, when it seemed a novelty; I climbed up on a stool from the main-level deck and could just peer over the edge of one of the nests to see three mottled-blue robin eggs. I thought them to be much bluer than the gallbladder, which is described in many surgical texts as "robin's egg blue." In more recent years the novelty has worn off and every fall I blast the condo project out into space with my gas-powered leaf blower.

It is springtime now, and Evie is visiting from Omaha. She is four years old and has a sister—her name is Gabby. I find myself at the back of our house in the approximate vicinity of where I would have fallen if the coefficient of static friction had not prevented my plunge from the third-story roof four years previously while unhooking the hornet-infested satellite dish. I am there to cut a few chives that Sue needs for dinner. I grab a fistful of the green spears of cellulose in my left hand, which I know are largely indigestible and therefore of little caloric content, and sharply snip them with the scissors in my right. I straighten up and turn back towards the house. The ground drops precipitously behind me and three stories of glass and wood rise before me and as always I feel a bit sheepish that only two people live in such a large building.

As I step to the wooden staircase that leads up to a separate landing, built solely for the purpose of exiting the garage through a back door, there is a frantic feathery burst of activity from the rafters of the upper-level deck, twenty feet to the right and two stories up. I see a gaggle of robins rocket into the trees, all but for one, which flutters down to the stairs in front of me. It chirps softly and waddles into the shadow of the stair above it.

I am immediately reminded of a movie that Sue and I watched just the previous week called *The Color of Paradise*, in which the first scene involved a blind boy, who is sitting on a park bench, waiting for his father to pick him up, when he hears a baby bird fall from its nest. With his sharply tuned sense of hearing the boy is able to follow the bird's plaintive chirps, climb the tree, at the base of which it lay, and gently place it back in its nest—aided only by his perception of sound and touch. It was quite a moving scene.

Right then, I decide that I too will replace the baby bird back in its nest, just like the little blind boy in the movie. It is surprisingly easy to pick baby-bird up. I hold his freshly feathered body in my right hand with his head protruding from the oval formed by my thumb and forefinger. He looks at me and opens his beak wide. I look back—*soon, baby-bird, soon.* I feel the heartbeat—about two hundred beats a minute, a gentle rapid tapping against the palm of my hand.

Inside the house, anxious to share my movie-like experience, I call out, "Evie … Gabby, look. Grandpa found a baby bird." I hold it out for them to see.

Evie wants to hold it, but I remember the previous summer when I gave her a frog from our pond and she squeezed it so hard that its eyes bugged out and its stomach telescoped out of its mouth. "Look, Grandpa. Little Froggy is sick," she said.

I'm not sure baby-bird would survive Evie's grip and so I say to her, "Little birdy is scared, Evie—why don't you just pet his head."

Evie pets baby-bird's head and coos, "It's okay, little birdy, it's okay—don't be scared." Gabby lightly touches the top of baby-bird's head with her finger, the nail painted a pastel purple, until the robin opens its beak, which causes Gabby to sharply withdraw her hand.

It is time. My heart swells with tenderness for baby-bird. I *am* the little blind boy from the movie, except that I can see. I climb the three-foot stepladder I placed next to the deck railing underneath the rafters of the third-story deck. I see a row of nests. I figure that any one will do.

My hand holding baby-bird is about three quarters of the way from the top of the deck rail to the rafters over my head while my other hand grasps one of the deck joists for balance. Evie, Gabby, and the rest of my family, drawn by the unfolding beneficent drama, watch expectantly. My heart swells further—like the Grinch's heart on Christmas Day when he decides to give the presents back. Baby-bird is nearly back in his nest. At that moment they strike.

The idyllic peace of the afternoon is shattered by the screeching of half a dozen robins that erupt from the canopy of leaves opposite the deck. Their feathers are fluffed out so that they are twice their normal size and I swear to God that they look like a flock of screaming eagles headed straight for my eyes. I jerk back from the nest and lose my balance. My right hand opens reflexively and baby-bird flies, straight and true, into the trees. With my right arm free I am able to keep myself from nose-diving over the deck rail on a familiar trajectory, and I am wishing that I at least had had the equanimity to yell—*Fly, baby-bird…Fly.*

#

I was sitting in church one Sunday morning not long ago, minding my own business, when suddenly a beautiful passage was thrust upon me. It happened to be the first reading of the lectionary. I know that the lectionary repeats every three years; the prodigal son, the "cast not the first stone," the "you saved the best wine for last" party, and so on. This one, however, I did not remember. It spoke of wisdom.

From Proverbs Chapter 8
(The Discourse of Wisdom), verses 22–31

> "The Lord begot me, the first-born of his ways,
> The forerunner of his prodigies of long ago;
> From of old I was poured forth,
> at the first, before the earth.
> When there were no depths I was brought forth,
> When there were no fountains or springs of
> water;
> Before the mountains were settled into place,
> Before the hills, I was brought forth;
> While as yet the earth and the fields were not
> made,
> Nor the first clods of the world.
> "When he established the heavens I was there,
> When he marked out the vault over the face of
> the deep;
> When he made firm the skies above,
> When he fixed fast the foundations of the earth;
> When he set for the sea its limit,

so that the waters should not transgress his
command;
Then was I beside him as his craftsman,
And I was his delight day by day,
Playing before him all the while,
Playing on the surface of his earth;
And I found delight in the sons of men."

The reason the above passage caught my eye is because
of the primordial role it assigns to wisdom, which I have
been thinking of as the awareness that is unique to us
alone in all the universe. The passage defines wisdom as
existing before all things, executed before the creation
of the universe. Although it speaks of wisdom as coming
from God, "The Lord begot me," I have trouble separat-
ing the two. Then I think of the wisdom of Newton—the
immortality of his thought, brought forth from a minute
collection of stardust, a jumble of electricity and space—
and I cannot help but think of the wisdom in each of
us as the embodiment of God on earth…"*And I found
delight in the sons of men.*"

And if you do not believe in a God as creator, that is
your choice, and I respect that; but then believe in this—
believe in wisdom, the freedom to choose, and the power
of positive thought and "to do good things."

It is finished.

You now know what you need to know to change
your life.

So…*Fly, dear reader…Fly.*

Finally, on the outside chance that you are a cheap bastard, standing in a bookstore and reading this last chapter to save yourself the discounted cover price of my book, you are probably thinking something along the lines of—*this is supposed to help me lose weight?* And you would be right. There wouldn't be that much meaning in these last few pages. Newton's third law of motion tells us that for every action there is an opposite and equal reaction. You need a *big* action. You need to be pushed from your current state of relativity. You need to change your frame of reference, and in order for me to start you on your way, I need to touch you, to flip a switch somewhere deep inside; and, for that to happen, you need to know a little about the universe.

Appendix

What the heck do I do now?

Okay. You've finished reading a long book and you may have a vague idea of what to do next, but you're not quite sure where to start, and the prospect of rereading the book would likely engender the same outcome as a narcoleptic sitting down in a La-Z-Boy to read *War and Peace* after lunch in a warm room; then this appendix is for you. Apart from realizing the importance of being open to the possibility of happiness, which is completely within your control, the emotionless, mechanical steps towards a positive change in your lifestyle are neither particularly long nor particularly complex, and most importantly, they make perfect sense and are backed up by the natural law of our beautifully mysterious universe. They are summarized as follows.

On being happy

Emotional health is an important part of making a positive change in your lifestyle. If I didn't think so, I wouldn't
have spent so much time on it. What I eventually wrote
represents less than half of what I put together initially
but I edited out quite a bit and overall, this was the most
difficult part for me, largely because the topic is very
subjective and means different things to different people. So, if you aren't happy yet, or aren't on your way to
being happy, perhaps there might be some utility in rereading the first pillar if you felt it at all helpful the first
time through.

On dieting

This is the easy part, and most simply stated is *honor
the first law of thermodynamics;* ultimately, at the end
of the day, it is always *calories in equals calories out.* All
you need to do is simply follow the rules. The first thing
to do is to know what your daily caloric intake is. The
detailed description is found in chapter twelve under
the subheading "Determining daily caloric need" and the
basic formula is body weight (lb.) multiplied by eleven.
Remember that the body weight represents your goal
after weight loss.

1. Count your calories: this means buying a scale,
    and a calorie-counter guide.
2. Record your calories: it does no good to count
    your calories if you are not going to record them.
    Write them down, every day on paper, or keep

a running total in an Excel spreadsheet, minimized at the bottom of your computer screen.
3. Honor portion size: by counting calories and
weighing your portions, this should be automatic.
4. Eat frequently (every 3–4 hours): note that I did
not say "Eat excessively." *Never ever* skip breakfast; by the time morning rolls around, your
body is already in the fasting mode and your
metabolic rate is depressed; you only compound
this by remaining in the fasting mode. Remember that eating causes DIT, which means that it
slightly raises your metabolic rate.

On macronutrients

1. Control carbohydrates: carbohydrates stimulate insulin secretion, and insulin suppresses
fat metabolism. Avoid high glycemic index carbohydrates found in refined sugars, soda pop,
sweets, white breads, pasta and corn. Ingested
carbohydrates as part of snacks or meals should
be low glycemic index and ideally balanced with
at least as much protein and fiber on a gram-for-
gram basis; that is to say, avoid snacks that are
(in total) more than 50 percent carbohydrate. At
the end of the day, at least while in the weight
loss phase, you should try to limit your carbohydrates to less than 30 percent of the total (ex.
about 150 grams for a 1,800 Cal/day diet). Even
if you don't, but still honor the first law, you will
lose weight; it is just that I am of the mind that
by controlling carbohydrates, and therefore
insulin, the weight loss process is facilitated.

2. Protein is good: it has the highest cost of DIT, it causes satiety, and it is a good source of energy that can be converted into glucose by the body. Low-fat sources of protein are better and allow you to eat more food, *which I always find helpful,* than higher-fat sources of protein.

3. Fat is good, too: especially those that I identified as "good fat," namely, those found in the Mediterranean diet such as olive and nut oils, as well as the omega-3 fatty acids. Fat is the most energy dense of the three macronutrients and if you eat more of it, you will eat less.

4. Bottom line: limit calories to daily requirement, control carbohydrates, eat whatever fat or protein you want that is left over within your daily requirement.

5. Do not take pills or have an operation without trying this first.

On exercise

1. Exercise six days out of the week: ideally for sixty minutes, and if not sixty, then thirty.

2. Exercise at low to moderate intensity: at this level, you are metabolizing primarily fat; if you exercise at a higher intensity (>60 percent max. heart rate) you will metabolize mostly stored glucose, until it runs out a couple of hours later.

3. Exercise in the morning (aerobic) before breakfast: or, if you have to eat, then eat a high-protein

breakfast with minimal low glycemic index carbohydrates, like eggs and ham, grapefruit, cottage cheese, whole wheat muffin with poached
egg and ham or cheese—you know what I man.

4. Avoid exercising after a higher-carbohydrate
    meal: because there will be a relative suppres-
    sion of the fat metabolism and you will burn
    mostly carbohydrate during your exercise ses-
    sion; but, if that is the only time you can exercise
    that day, then exercise, most definitely.

5. Eat after exercising: this means a mid-morning
    or mid-afternoon snack, if not one of the major
    meals of the day. If you are eating something six
    times a day, as you should be, this is not difficult
    to do.

6. Resistance training: two of the six days should
    be reserved for resistance training. The resis-
    tance training program in the appendix is an
    example, but any program you find elsewhere
    should work just as well as long as you follow the
    general guidelines in the appendix.

7. Aerobic training: the remaining four days of our
    six should be spent on aerobic training, and it
    would be helpful to eventually work in one epi-
    sode of endurance training, which simply means
    prolonged aerobic activity of 1.5 to 2.0 hours.
    This allows for a prolonged period of fat metabo-
    lism (as long as it's low to moderate activity)
    and if this happens a lot, your body just might
    become that much better at metabolizing fat.

8. Do not worry about exercise-specific nutrition,
    unless you are an elite athlete, and if you are,

and have still read my book, then *thank you for your kind attention.*

Wow. Did it really take me over three hundred pages just to say that? *Yes.* Because, now you not only know what to do—you know *why* to do it. I am not just pulling this stuff out of my you-know-where. I am pulling this stuff out of evidence-based science and the natural physical laws of our universe. I truly hope that you understand that, and appreciate the *why* and the *how* of weight loss and the *importance of being happy.*

Resistance training

As I said before, the most important thing about resistance training is that it's not so important what you do as it is that you actually do it. The general guidelines for the recreational weight lifter are as follows:

1. Exercise muscle groups no more than two times per week.
2. Perform only one to two sets of 10–12 repetitions of each type.
3. It is more important to increase resistance than it is to increase repetitions.
4. The weight should be such that you come close to muscle failure towards the end of the repetitions (you couldn't lift just one more time).
5. Don't forget the largest muscles (legs) because they have the largest potential for increase in lean muscle mass and thereby increase in metabolic rate.

For the purposes of general fitness, increase in lean muscle mass and improved bone density and joint strength, there is no need to exercise each individual muscle group every second or third day by lifting multiple sets in multiple repetitions over the course of two to three hours. It is much easier than that; in fact, there is little improvement in taking the time to do two sets of 10–12 repetitions over the time spent on doing only one, as long as that first set is performed to muscle failure.

Now, I am not suggesting that after a lifetime, or at least several years, of overweight*ness* or obesity, compounded by a sedentary lifestyle, you immediately begin lifting to muscle failure. If you do that you'll likely strain a muscle or tear a rotator cuff or worse. For the first week or two I'd suggest lighter weights to perhaps 80 percent effort, until you become used to the routine and have a better idea of your limits.

The final caveat is to never forget to stretch prior to (and following) any type of exercise, but this is particularly important with resistance training. This doesn't need to be difficult or time-consuming. I typically take about five to ten minutes between the pre- and post-exercise stretching.

Beginning on the next page, I illustrate what I've come to refer to as the "Phalanx" in the text of the third pillar of the DTOE. This largely covers the upper body, but could be supplemented by other exercises if you have the equipment, the time, or the desire.

The first series exercises the deltoid muscles (shoulders) and involves ten repetitions of three movements, each side simultaneously. I illustrate the start and end of each movement for all of the exercises.

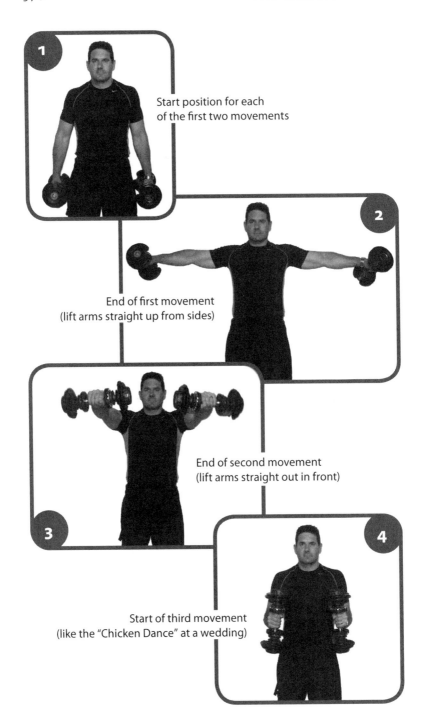

Start position for each
of the first two movements

End of first movement
(lift arms straight up from sides)

End of second movement
(lift arms straight out in front)

Start of third movement
(like the "Chicken Dance" at a wedding)

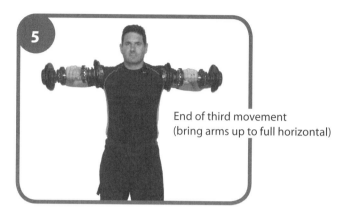

End of third movement
(bring arms up to full horizontal)

This next set involves six movements of ten repetitions all done alternating, except for the last one. These exercise chest, back, lateral abdominal, and arm muscles.

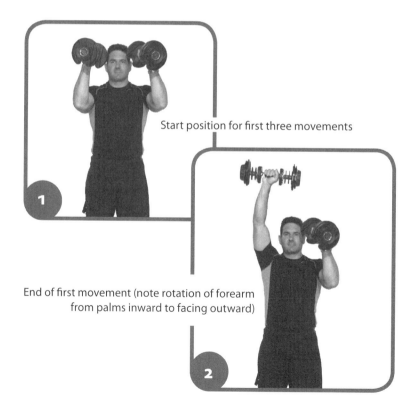

Start position for first three movements

End of first movement (note rotation of forearm from palms inward to facing outward)

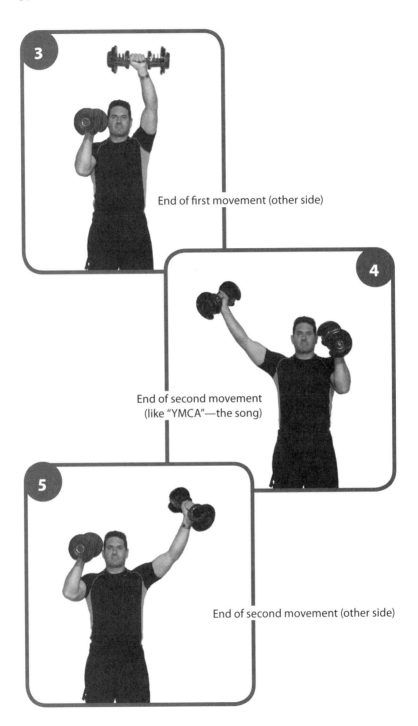

End of first movement (other side)

End of second movement
(like "YMCA"—the song)

End of second movement (other side)

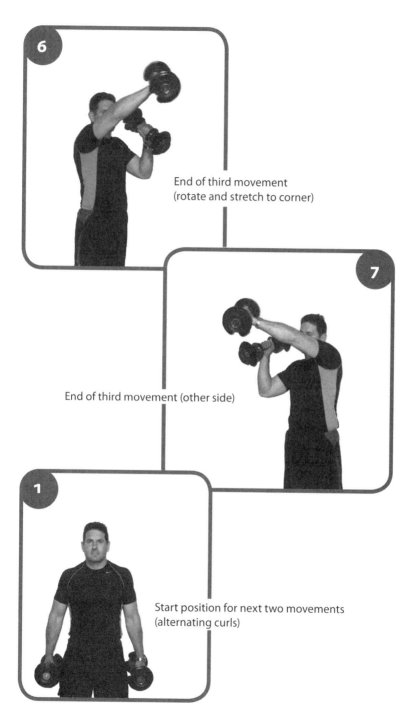

End of third movement
(rotate and stretch to corner)

End of third movement (other side)

Start position for next two movements
(alternating curls)

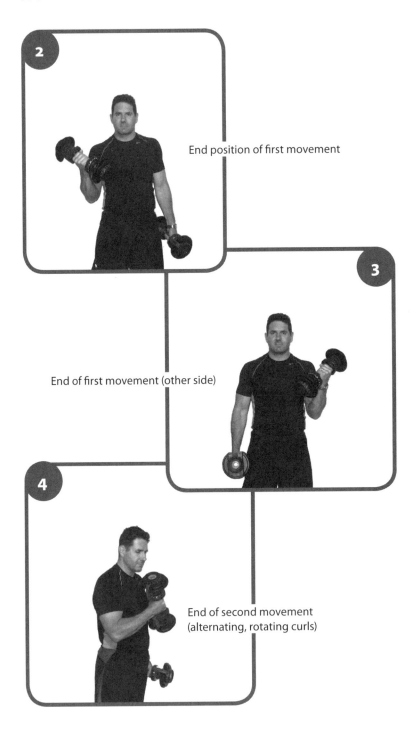

2 End position of first movement

3 End of first movement (other side)

4 End of second movement (alternating, rotating curls)

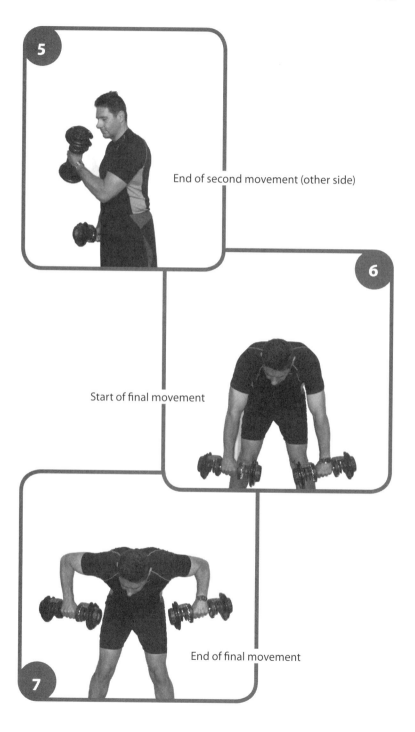

5

End of second movement (other side)

6

Start of final movement

End of final movement

7

This completes the official repetitions of the Phalanx, which should only take about ten minutes per set. As part of these exercises I mix in 45 push-ups with my feet balanced on a Pilates ball, and ten alternating butterfly lifts on a back bench—per *each set of the Phalanx.*

As we are interested in balance, let us not forget core strength and our leg muscles. This will round out the remaining time in our hour or so of resistance training. Again, it doesn't matter so much what you do here, as long as you do something. This would be a nice place for a Pilates core strength routine. I will typically do eighty repetitions (one side) of various abdominal crunches/ sit-ups, with at least half involving rotation.

To the uninitiated, this seems like a lot; and to the athlete, this seems like not much at all. As everything, it is all relative to your particular frame of reference. All of my resistance exercises that I do, when I do them all, which includes some leg exercises, take me about an hour and twenty minutes. There are some weeks where I get lazy and only do the resistance training once, which will keep me from detraining.

All I would suggest is that you start slow, with lighter weights, and gradually work up from there. After a few weeks you will start feeling much better and will be thankful that you started. It will be just one of many positive alternate realities that you chose. Good luck.

When I just gotta eat

It is easy, most of the time, to plan your meals and to have the required ingredients available. What might be more difficult to deal with are those times between meals when you're starving, or you just gotta eat *some-*

thing. The following list is certainly not inclusive, nor is it even recommended. It is simply a short list of foods I try to have available. As long as you do a little research into the various macronutrient proportions, and qualities, of the foods that you like, you will develop your very own list of "comfort" foods that are appropriate and consistent with the general principles of the DTOE. Remember that this is what I eat, and I am a big guy, even when at an appropriate BMI. My daily requirements are 2,400 Calories; so, the below might not be in appropriate portions for some sweet young thing with a daily caloric requirement of 1,500 Calories.

1. Whole grain wraps: I buy these things by the gross. Each wrap has 100 Calories, and I will put peanut butter (1 Tbsp—80 Cal) and either sugar-free jelly (10 Cal) or ⅛ cup dried cherries (40 Cal) on it and roll it up, and then I eat it.

2. Meal bars: I buy various brands, with the only requirement being less than 250 Calories/bar and at least ten (preferably more) grams of protein. Oftentimes I will add about 60–70 Calories of peanut butter and dried cherries if it really is replacing a meal. If I'm having a long day, I'll have the same thing for an afternoon snack.

3. Snack bars: again, I buy various brands, with the only requirement being less than 160 Calories/bar and at least five (preferably more) grams of protein. I don't eat this too often, but Sue does (since she's a sweet young thing).

4. Low-fat cottage cheese: is a great comfort food or snack to have around if you like it. It can be

seasoned, or eaten with fruit. It has three times as much protein as carbohydrate.

5. Pickled things: herring, artichoke hearts, and other less palatable animal parts that are probably more guy-specific, like gizzards, pork hocks, etc.

My typical breakfast

One third of a cup of Egg Beaters (45 Cal) in a microwave egg-poaching thing that Sue picked up one day; I also add two thin slices of Canadian bacon (25 Cal), and three large sliced olives (40 Cal) before popping it in the microwave for 40 seconds; then I add a sprinkle of shredded cheese (50 Cal), poke it with a spoon and give it another 40 seconds of radio-frequency ablation. I stick my poached egg conglomeration in a whole grain "light" English muffin (100 Cal) with low-fat margarine (20 Cal), and then I eat it. Usually I'll have some fruit as well, like a grapefruit, strawberries or an apple. The total caloric cost, other than the fruit, is 280 Calories, and 40 of those are the olives, which some people don't care for.

Sue's typical breakfast

Sue's breakfast isn't as protein-intensive as mine, but it works for her. She'll have the same muffin, sans butter, and plain yogurt mixed with sugar-free jelly and a pack of Splenda. But, her yogurt is "special." Let me explain. She puts a large container of plain yogurt in a strainer that fits into a bowl—this allows the water to drain out and what is left is a stiff, almost like cream cheese, yogurt. One half of a cup of yogurt (50 Cal) on the English muffin (100 Cal) and the sugar-free jelly (10 Cal) yields a total of 160 Cal for breakfast, in addition to a serving of fruit.

Yogurt has a little more carbohydrate than protein, so in someone trying to exert a tighter control on their carbo-hydrates, some variation of my breakfast would be better.

As I said, these foods that I eat comprise a short list, but there are many different foods and snacks that would be consistent with the recommendations that I have put forth. Please do some homework and research different foods and snacks that you think would work for you—until you do, please, help yourself to some pickled pork hocks.

Healthy whole foods

Remember—moderation and balance—the below should represent portions of your diet. The calories still count, as do the carbohydrates (especially fruit). Also, remember that the glycemic index of food is lowered with mixed meals, generous in fiber.

Whole grains: whole wheat bread, wraps, pasta, high-fiber cereal, oatmeal, wild rice, brown rice

Beans/legumes: chickpeas, black, white, kidney, lima, butter, lentils

Vegetables: broccoli, cauliflower, cabbage, kale, Brussels sprouts, spinach, lettuce, tomatoes

Vegetables and fruits rich in vitamin A: carrots, sweet potato, squash, apricots, mangoes, papayas, passion fruit

Flaxseed, nuts

Berries: strawberries, raspberries, blueberries, blackberries

Fruits: grapefruit, oranges, apples

Soy products

Garlic, green tea, red wine

Spices/Herbs: rosemary, turmeric, chili peppers.

Glossary

adenovirus   the class of viruses associated with the common cold; the subtype Ad-36 has been linked to obesity.

adipocyte   a cell that synthesizes and stores fat in the form of triglycerides.

aerobic metabolism   the molecular breakdown of nutrients for the purpose of energy utilization, in the presence of oxygen.

amalgam   a blending or combination of two or more substances.

anabolic   the process of building up, generally in regard to biological tissue.

anaerobic metabolism   the molecular breakdown of nutrients for the purpose of energy utilization, in the absence of oxygen.

android obesity   the type of obesity more commonly associated with men; central or visceral obesity; "apple shape."

ascites   the presence of fluid inside the peritoneal cavity (intra-abdominal).

atom   the smallest unit of structure of an element; composed of a nucleus surrounded by electrons in orbital shell(s); the atom is 99.999 percent space.

atomic number   is equal to the number of protons in the nucleus.

atomic weight   more accurately called the atomic mass as it represents a ratio of the average mass of an atom to $\frac{1}{12}$ the mass of carbon; the number is listed on the periodic table.

Avogadro's number   is a constant that represents the number of atoms in exactly 12 grams of carbon-12, or one mole of a substance; 6.022×10^{23}.

bariatric surgery   the surgery of obesity.

basal metabolic rate (BMR)   the minimal level of metabolism necessary for biological processes; measured after twelve hours of fasting and at rest.

Big Bang   the beginning of the universe, which theoretically erupted from an infinitesimally small point of unimaginable heat and density.

Body mass index (BMI)   a standardized measurement to define underweight, normal weight, overweight and obesity; based on an individual's height and weight.

bosons   particles of matter that have zero or whole spin numbers, such as the photon; are not excluded by Pauli's exclusion principle.

calorie   a unit of energy; the amount of energy required to raise the temperature of 1 gram of water by 1 degree Celsius.

calorimeter   an apparatus used to measure the energy of a substance obtained from its complete combustion.

catabolic   energy production obtained from the breakdown of biological or organic fuel.

Centers for Disease Control and Prevention (CDC)   a
sixty-year-old federal agency dedicated to protect-
ing health and quality of life; budgeted 8.8 billion
dollars in 2009.

central obesity   also referred to as visceral obesity;
refers to accumulation of fat around the center of
the body and specifically intra-peritoneally (inside
the abdomen), where it surrounds and accumulates
in the organs; more common in android obesity.

Copenhagen interpretation   an interpretation of quantum mechanics in which everything is based on
probability; somewhat synonymous with the uncertainty principle.

daguerreotype   the earliest photographs in the 1800s;
utilized silver-coated plates.

diabetes, type 1   also known as juvenile-onset diabetes, although adults can suffer from this as well;
characterized by an inability of the pancreas to
secrete enough insulin, resulting in elevated blood
sugar levels.

diabetes, type 2   also known as adult onset diabetes;
in the early stages is non–insulin dependent and
treatable with diet and medications, in later stages
becomes insulin dependent; characterized by tissue
resistance to the insulin—in the initial stages the
pancreas secretes normal to elevated levels of insulin but because of the tissue resistance, blood sugars
remain high.

diet-induced thermogenesis   refers to the elevation of
the metabolic rate with the ingestion of macronutrients; the elevation is most with protein and the least
with fat.

double-slit lamp experiment   one of the most famous
and beautiful experiments in physics which proves
the duality of light and matter; please refer to text.

electromagnetic force   one of the four fundamental forces of the universe related to the electrical attraction of electrons to the atomic nucleus;
exemplified by the daily use of electricity in our
lives.

electron   a subatomic particle, a fermion, which has
a negative charge and occupies a specific space
around the atomic nucleus.

element   a substance composed of similar atoms that
cannot be broken down any further; there are 92
naturally occurring elements on earth.

ephemeral   momentary or transient and leaving no
trace of its existence.

epidemiology   the study of the cause and transmission
of disease within a population.

Eucharist prayer   also known as the Anaphora, which
is the most solemn part of the Christian Mass, during which the offerings of bread and wine are conse-
crated as the body and blood of Christ.

**excess post-exercise oxygen consumption
(EPOC)**   refers to the extra oxygen that is used
following exercise and that persists for a period
of hours following exercise; is associated with an
elevation in the metabolic rate; most significant following periods of submaximal or maximal exertion.

fermion   elementary particles of matter, including
electrons, protons, and neutrons; particles with
whole spin numbers and subject to Pauli's exclusion
principle.

first law of thermodynamics   pertains to the universal law of the conservation of energy: energy can be neither created nor destroyed.

flagitiousness   a complicated word for "sin."

fundamental force   there are four fundamental forces in our universe; electromagnetic, strong nuclear, weak nuclear, and gravity.

globesity   a play on the words "globe" and "obesity" to reflect the worldwide problem of obesity.

gluconeogenesis   the process of synthesis of glucose.

glucose   a six-carbon sugar that is the ultimate basic unit of all ingested carbohydrates utilized for energy or stored as glycogen or converted into fat.

glycemic index   refers to the rate of absorption of a carbohydrate; a slower rate of absorption, "low glycemic index," is generally more desirable than a higher rate of absorption, "high-glycemic index."

gram calorie   a unit of energy; the amount of energy required to raise the temperature of 1 gram of water by 1 degree Celsius; distinguished from the nutritional calorie, which is 1,000 gram calories, or a kilocalorie.

grand unification theory   refers to a unified theory under which both the classical physics of Einstein and Newton (gravity) and quantum mechanics will both fit.

gynoid obesity   the type of obesity most commonly associated with women; peripheral obesity; "pear shape."

hermaphroid obesity   a word I made up that implies obesity with equal amounts of android and gynoid contributions.

homily   the sermon (lecture) that follows the Gospel
reading; precedes the offertory.

id   from Freudian psychoanalytical theory; the portion of the consciousness involved in instinctive
impulses and pleasure seeking; the other components are the ego and superego.

inflammation   the hallmark of tissue injury represented by redness, heat, swelling and pain.

insulin   a hormone produced by the pancreatic islet
cells and released into the blood in response to
carbohydrate or glucose ingestion; involved in the
regulation of blood glucose; an anabolic hormone
that suppresses fat metabolism and encourages fat
storage.

interference pattern   the pattern demonstrated by
wave behavior when series of waves "interfere"
with one another—where two crests meet, there is
an especially high wave; where a crest and a trough
meet, there is a cancellation.

joule   unit of measure for energy, more commonly used
in Europe. $1 J = 1 kg \times m^2/s^2$; 4.2 joules = 1 calorie

kinetic energy   energy in motion; a 1 kg weight falling
from a height is expending kinetic energy during
its fall; the kinetic energy is equal to the potential
energy of that 1 kg weight when at rest at some
height above the surface of the earth; in accordance
with the law of the conservation of energy, when the
1 kg weight strikes the earth and comes to a stop the
kinetic energy is converted to heat and the mechanical energy of the displacement of some amount of
the earth.

kwashiorkor malnutrition   malnutrition caused by an
inadequate intake of protein.

leptin   a hormone produced by fat cells that is released into the blood and acts on the hypothalamus of the brain to indicate satiety; in obesity, the tissues can become resistant to the persistently elevated levels of leptin and the sensation of satiety is blunted.

Little Boy   the name given to the nuclear bomb dropped on Hiroshima; a "gun type" nuclear device in which two lumps of uranium-235 were slammed together, triggering a chain reaction of nuclear fission (splitting).

macronutrient   refers to classes of food that are metabolized in a similar fashion; fat, protein, and carbohydrate.

many worlds theory   a theory within the realm of quantum mechanics which supposes that there are an infinite number of alternate universes that branch off such that every possible outcome to every possible event occurs in some alternate reality; we can only be aware of the events in our own reality.

Mendelian   refers to the genetic transmission of traits from parent to child; the laws of inheritance were first derived by a 19th-century monk, Gregor Mendel.

metabolic syndrome   a prediabetic condition characterized by glucose intolerance, hypertension, obesity, high triglycerides/cholesterol, pro-inflammatory state.

molecule   the smallest unit of a substance that consists of one or more atoms held together by the electromagnetic force of chemical energy.

morbidity   the presence of illness or a disease, or a complication thereof.

morphology   the structure and form of an organism or a part of an organism.

mortality   death.

National Heart, Lung, and Blood Institute (NHLBI)
focuses on research into the treatment of diseases of
the heart, lungs, and blood; a federal health agency
with an annual budget of 3 billion dollars that falls
under the jurisdiction of the National Institutes of
Health (NIH), with an annual budget of nearly 30
billion dollars.

neutron   a subatomic particle (fermion) that has zero
charge and resides in the nucleus of an atom.

nucleus   the center of the atom and consists of subatomic particles (neutron, proton, etc.), all held
together by the immensely powerful strong nuclear
force.

nutritional calorie   please see "gram calorie."

offertory   that part of the church service where the
gifts and bread and wine are brought to the front of
the church.

omentum   refers to a fatty layer of the abdominal lining (peritoneum) that hangs down from the stomach
and covers the intestine.

orbital shell   refers to the spherical space that an electron inhabits around the nucleus of an atom; dia-
grammatically is represented as a planetary orbit
around a central body (nucleus).

oxidation   a chemical reaction in which oxygen is
added to an element or a compound; in the process
of oxidation, electrons are lost from the chemical
element or compound.

pannus   the pendulous belly composed of peripheral
fat outside of the peritoneal cavity that hangs down
past the waistline.

periodic table   a table of all known elements, consisting of 117 elements, 94 of these naturally occurring on earth.

peripheral obesity   the accumulation of fat in peripheral tissues; see "central obesity"; more common in gynoid obesity.

photon   an elemental particle (boson), with zero charge and zero mass; a particle of light which travels at light speed and is therefore timeless.

physiology   the study of the function of living things from the cellular level to the macro level, including metabolism, reproduction and organ systems.

Planck's constant   named after Max Planck, who was an early pioneer of quantum theory; measured in units of energy multiplied by time (joule seconds); an unbelievably small number denoted by $\hbar$, and on the scale of 10^{-34}.

potential energy   see "kinetic energy."

pro-inflammatory   indicates a sensitization to the inflammatory state (pre-inflammatory); see "inflammation."

proton   a subatomic particle (fermion) of a positive charge and mass that resides within the nucleus of an atom.

quantum mechanics   the set of principles and universal truths underlying all physical systems at the elemental scale (atomic, molecular).

quantum numbers   a set of four numbers that specify the approximate location and momentum or energy of the electrons of atoms.

quarks   some of the smallest elementary particles that have a fraction of a whole charge and mass;

quarks make up the particles of matter, such as a
proton, which is composed of three of the six types
of quarks.

resting daily energy expenditure similar to basal
metabolic rate (BMR); only requires four hours of
fast and typically is within a few percentage points
of the BMR; easier to measure.

set point theory the theory that an individual's weight
is "set" and that the metabolic rate will slow down
or speed up to maintain weight at the set point; has
been disproven.

strong nuclear force the strongest of the four fundamental forces that holds the subatomic particles of
the nucleus together; remember that the electrical
tendency is for the like, positive charges of the protons to repel.

theory of everything see grand unification theory.

uncertainty principle analogous to the Copenhagen
interpretation.

Unna boot a medicated-paste wrap that is applied to
the lower leg for compression and the treatment of
leg ulcers secondary to venous stasis disease.

venous stasis disease a common condition of obesity
in which there is an elevated venous pressure in the
legs that results in chronic swelling and weeping of
fluid into the soft tissues and eventual skin breakdown and discoloration and woodiness.

visceral obesity see "central obesity."

weak nuclear force one of the four fundamental
forces; represents nuclear decay (radiation).

white adipose tissue simply another name for fat
stores; acts as a gland that releases leptin and the

chemical mediators of inflammation; implicated in the pro-inflammatory state.

World Health Organization   an international organization responsible for providing global health assistance; within the United Nations System of Organizations; annual budget of about 5 billion dollars funded by member nations.

References

1   Centers for Disease Control and Prevention. [Online] www.cdc.gov:80/nchs/Default.htm.

2   World Health Organization. [Online] www.who.int /mediacentre/factsheets/fs311/en/index.html.

3   National Institutes of Health. [Online] http://win .niddk.nih.gov/statistics/index.htm.

4   National Heart, Lung, and Blood Institute. [Online] www.nhlbi.nih.gov/guidelines/obesity/e_txtbk /ratnl/213.htm.

5   *Clinical Guidelines on the Identification, Evaluation, and Treatment of Overweight and Obesity in Adults: The Evidence Report.* National Heart Lung and Blood Institute. [Online] 1998. www.nhlbi.nih.gov /guidelines/obesity/ob_gdlns.htm.

6   Circulating mononuclear cells in the obese are in a proinflammatory state. Husam G, et al. 110, s.l.: *Circulation*, 2004, pp. 1564–1571.

7 Metabolic syndrome and cardiovascular disease. Qing Q, et al. 44, s.l.: *Ann Clin Biochem*, pp. 232–263.

8 Recent advances in the relationship between obesity, inflammation, and insulin resistance. Bastard J, et al. 1, s.l.: *Eur Cytokine Netw*, March 2006, Vol. 17 n, pp. 4–12.

9 The metabolic consequences of childhood obesity. Weiss R, et al. 3, s.l.: *Best Pract Res Clin Endocrinol Metab,* 2005, Vol. 19, pp. 404–419.

10 Cause-specific excess deaths associated with underweight, overweight and obesity. Flegal K, et al. 17, s.l.: *JAMA*, 2007, Vol. 298, pp. 2028–2037.

11 Review article: nutrition, obesity and colorectal cancer. Johnson I, et al. s.l.: *Aliment Pharmacol Ther*, 2007, Vol. 26, pp. 161–181.

12 Heart scan blog. blogspot.com. [Online] http://heartscanblog.blogspot.com/2006/09/are-you-skinny-fat-person.html.

13 True Star Health. [Online] www.truestarhealth .com/members/cm_archives14_ML3_P1_A11.html.

14 McArdle, Katch, Katch. *Exercise Physiology*, Sixth Edition. s.l.: Lippincott Williams & Wilkins, 2007. p. 865.

15 McArdle, Katch, Katch. *Exercise Physiology*, Sixth Edition. s.l.: Lippincott Williams & Wilkins, 2007. p. 839.

16 The response to long-term overfeeding in identical twins. Bouchard C, et al. s.l.: *N Engl J Med*, 1990, Vol. 322, pp. 1477–1482.

17 Obesity—is it a genetic disorder. Loos R, Bouchard C. s.l.: *J Intern Med*, 2003, Vol. 254, pp. 401–425.

18 Inheritance of the amount and distribution of

human body fat. Bouchard C, et al. 205, s.l.: *Int J Obes*, 1988, Vol. 12.

19 Leptin: obesity, diabetes and other peripheral effects—a review. Moran O, Phillip M. s.l.: *Pediatr Diabetes*, 2003, Vol. 4, pp. 101–109.

20 Mechanisms of leptin action and leptin resistance. Myers MG, et al. s.l.: *Annu Rev Physiol*, 2008, Vol. 70, pp. 537–556.

21 McArdle, Katch, Katch. *Exercise Physiology*, Sixth Edition. s.l.: Lippincott Williams & Wilkins, 2007. p. 843.

22 Free-living activity energy expenditure in women successful and unsuccessful at maintaining a normal body weight. Weinsier R, et al. s.l.: *Am J Clin Nutr*, 2002, Vol. 75, pp. 499–504.

23 New data challenge popular set point theory of obesity—physical activity seems key. Jancin B. s.l.: *OB/GYN News*, 2003.

24 Human adenovirus-36 is associated with increased body weight and paradoxical reduction of serum lipids. Atkinson RL, et al. 3, s.l.: *Int J Obes (Lond)*, 2005, Vol. 29, pp. 281–286.

25 Adipogenic human adenovirus Ad-36 induces commitment, differentiation, and lipid accumulation in human adipose-derived stem cells. Pasarica M, Mashtalir N, et al. 4, April 2008, *Stem Cells*, Vol. 26, pp. 969–978.

26 Human adenovirus Ad-36 induces adipogenesis via its E4 orf-1 gene. Rogers PM, et al. s.l.: *Int J Obes (Lond)*, 2008, Vol. 32, pp. 397–406.

27 Feynman R, Leighton, Sands. *The Feynman Lectures on Physics*. s.l.: Pearson Addison Wesley, 2006. pp. 4–8. Vol. 1.

28 Rhoades R. *The Making of the Atomic Bomb.* s.l.: Simon & Schuster, 1986. pp. 700–714.

29 Taylor, I (Cambridge). PhysLink.com. [Online] www.physlink.com/education/askexperts/ae329 .cfm.

30 Big bang theory under fire. Mitchel W. 2, s.l.: *Physics Essays*, June 1997, Vol. 10.

31 Feynman R. *QED: The Strange Theory of Light and Matter.* s.l.: Princeton University Press, 2006.pp. 131–132.

32 McArdle, Katch, Katch. *Exercise Physiology*, Sixth Edition. s.l.: Lippincott Williams & Wilkins, 2007. pp. 140–145.

33 McArdle, Katch, Katch. *Exercise Physiology*, Sixth Edition. s.l.: Lippincott Williams & Wilkins, 2007. p. 27.

34 Msn.com. Moneycentral. [Online] http://articles .moneycentral.msn.com/SavingandDebt /ConsumerActionGuide/WhatDoesItCost ToDrop30Pounds.aspx.

35 Energy metabolism and obesity. Goran M. 2, s.l.: *Med Clin North Am*, March 2000, Vol. 34.

36 Strength training increases resting metabolic rate and norepinephrine levels in healthy 50–65 yr-old men. Pratley R, et al. 133, s.l.: *J Appl PHysiol*, 1994, Vol. 73.

37 Differences in daily energy expenditure in lean and obese women: the role of posture allocation. Johannsen D, et al. s.l.: *Obesity*, 2008, Vol. 16, pp. 34–39.

38 Diet induced thermogenesis measured over 24 h in a respiration chamber: effect of diet composition.

Westerterp KR, Wilson SA, Rolland V. 3, s.l.: *Int J Obes Relat Metab Disord*, 1999, Vol. 23, pp. 287–292.

39 Influence of autonomic nervous system on nutrient-induced thermogenesis in humans. Acheson KJ. 4, s.l.: *Nutrition*, 1993, Vol. 9, pp. 373–380.

40 Diet induced thermogenesis. Westerterp K. 5, August 18, 2004, *Nutr Metab (Lond)*, Vol. 1.

41 Gluttony 2: thermogenesis in overeating man. Miller DS, et al. s.l.: *Am J Clin Nutr*, 1967, Vol. 20, p. 1223.

42 Multivitamin use and risk of cancer and cardiovascular disease in the Women's Health Initiative cohorts. Neuhouser ML, Wassertheil-Smoller S, et al. 3, s.l.: *Arch Intern Med*, February 2009, Vol. 169, pp. 294–304.

43 Pharmacotherapy for obesity. Neff L, Aronne L. 6, s.l.: *Curr Atheroscler Rep,* 2007, Vol. 9, pp. 454–462.

44 Consumersearch.com. [Online] www.consumer search.com/www/health_and_fitness/diet-pills /review.html.

45 Dietary supplements for body-weight reduction: a systematic review. Pittler MH, Ernst E. 4, s.l.: *Am J Clin Nutr*, 2004, Vol. 79, pp. 529–536.

46 Mayoclinic.com. [Online] www.mayoclinic.com /health/weight-loss/HQ01160.

47 Availability of weight-loss supplements: results of an audit of retail outlets in a southeastern city. Sharpe PA, Granner ML, et al. 12, s.l.: *J Am Diet Assoc*, December 2006, Vol. 106, pp. 2045–2051.

48 Effect of conjugated linoleic acid on body composition in mice. Park Y, Albright KJ, et al. 8, August 1997, *Lipids*, Vol. 32, pp. 853–858.

49 Anti-obesity and anti-diabetic effects of CL316,243,
a highly specific beta 3-adrenoceptor agonist,
in Otsuka Long-Evans Tokushima Fatty rats:
induction of uncoupling protein and activation of
glucose transporter 4 in white fat. Umekawa T,
Yoshida T, et al. 4, April 1997, *Eur J Endocrinol*, Vol.
136, pp. 362–365.

50 Conjugated linoleic acid supplementation for 1 y
reduces body fat mass in healthy overweight
humans. Gaullier JM, Halse J, et al. 6, June 2004, *Am
J Clin Nutr*, Vol. 79, pp. 1118–1125.

51 Conjugated linoleic acid supplementation for 1 y
does not prevent weight or body fat regain. Larsen
TM, Toubro S, et al. 3, March 2006, Vol. 83, pp.
606–612.

52 Green tea extract thermogenesis-induced weight
loss by epigallocatechin gallate inhibition of cate-
chol-*O*-methyltransferase. Shixian Q, VanCrey B, et
al. 4, Winter 2006, *J Med Food*, Vol. 9, pp. 451–458.

53 Green tea reduces body fat accretion caused by
high-fat diet in rats through beta-adrenoceptor
activation of thermogenesis in brown adipose tissue. Choo JJ. 11, November 2003, *J Nutr Biochem*,
Vol. 14, pp. 671–676.

54 Effect of green tea on resting energy expenditure
and substrate oxidation during weight loss in
overweight females. Diepvens K, Kovacs EM, et al.
6, December 2005, *Br J Nutr*, Vol. 94, pp. 1026–1034.

55 Efficacy of 12 weeks supplementation of a botani-
cal extract-based weight loss formula on body
weight, body composition and blood chemistry in
healthy, overweight subjects—a randomized double-blind placebo controlled clinical trial. Opala T,

Rzymski P, et al. 8, August 30, 2006, *Eur J Med Res*, Vol. 11, pp. 343–350.

56 Increased ATP content/production in the hypothalamus may be a signal for energy-sensing of satiety: studies of the anorectic mechanism of a plant steroidal glycoside. MacLean DB, Luo LG. September 10, 2004, *Brain Res*, Vol. 1020 (1–2), pp. 1–11.

57 Telegraph.co.uk. [Online] www.telegraph.co.uk/finance/2859230/Pfizer-hands-Phytopharms-drug-back.html.

58 Chromium picolinate supplementation in women: effects on body weight, composition, and iron status. Lukaski HC, Siders WA, et al. 3, March 2007, *Nutrition*, Vol. 23, pp. 187–195.

59 The effect of chromium picolinate on muscular strength and body composition in women athletes. Livolsi JM, Adams GM, et al. 2, May 2001, *J Strength Cond Res*, Vol. 15, pp. 161–166.

60 Effects of resistance training and chromium picolinate on body composition and skeletal muscle in older men. Campbell WW, Joseph LJ, et al. 1, January 1999, *J Appl Physiol*, Vol. 86, pp. 29–39.

61 Effect of Lean System 7 on metabolic rate and body composition. Zenk JL, et al. 2005, *Nutrition*, Vol. 21, pp. 179–185.

62 Effects of bariatric surgery on mortality in Swedish obese subjects. Sjöström L, et al. August 2007, *N Engl J Med*, Vol. 357, pp. 741–752.

63 Convergence of body mass with aging: the longitudinal interrelationship of health, weight, and survival. Yang Z, et al. July 1, 2008, *Econ Hum Biol*.

64 Cost-effectiveness of gastric bypass for severe obe-

sity. Craig BM, et al. 2002, *Am J Med*, Vol. 113, pp. 491–498.

65 Current estimates of the economic cost of obesity in the United States. Wolf AM, et al. 1998, *Obes Res*, Vol. 6, pp. 97–106.

66 Guyton AC. *Textbook of Medical Physiology*, Seventh Edition. s.l.: Saunders, 1986. Chap. 67,68,73,78.

67 Soft drink consumption and risk of developing cardiometabolic risk factors and the metabolic syndrome in middle-aged adults in the community. Dhingra R, et al. 5, July 2007, *Epidemiology*, Vol. 116, pp. 480–488.

68 Diet soda intake and risk of incident metabolic syndrome and type 2 diabetes in the MESA. Nettleton JA, et al. Jan 16, 2009, *Diabetes Care*. Online.

69 The effect of artificial sweetener on insulin secretion. Liang Y, et al. 7, July 1987, *Horm Metab Res*, Vol. 19, pp. 285–289.

70 The anti-inflammatory effect of exercise: its role in diabetes and cardiovascular disease control. Pedersen B. 2006, *Essays Biochem*, Vol. 42, pp. 105–17.

71 Optimizing fat oxidation through exercise and diet. Achten J, et al. 2004, *Nutrition*, Vol. 20, pp. 716–727.

72 Postexercise nutrient intake timing in humans is critical to recovery of leg glucose and protein homeostasis. Levenhagen D, Gresham J, et al. 2001, *Am J Physiol Endocrinol Metab*, Vol. 280, pp. E982–E993.

73 Regulation of muscle glycogen repletion, muscle protein synthesis and repair following exercise.

Ivy J. 2004, *Journal of Sports Science and Medicine,* Vol. 3, pp. 132–138.

74 Effects of exercise intensity and duration on the excess post-exercise oxygen consumption. LaForgia J, et al. 12, December 2006, *J Sports Sci,* Vol. 24, pp. 1247–1264.

75 Exercise training and nutritional supplementation for physical frailty in very elderly people. Fiatarone MA, et al. 1994, *N Engl J Med,* Vol. 330, p. 1769.

Reading list

In addition to the bibliography I would like to acknowledge a "reading list" of books that have contributed to my personal growth. The list is not inclusive or in any particular order, other than the approximate order in which I read them, but these works are the ones that come to mind. I am indebted to the brilliance of each of these authors, without which little of what I have written would have been possible.

1 Brian Greene. *The Elegant Universe.* Random House. 2000.
2 John Gribbin. *In Search of Schrödinger's Cat: Quantum Physics and Reality.* Bantam Books. 1984.
3 John Gribbin. *Schrödinger's Kittens and the Search for Reality: Solving the Quantum Mysteries.* Back Bay Books. 1996.
4 William Shakespeare. *Hamlet.* Washington Square Press. 2003.

5　Walter Isaacson. *Einstein: His Life and Universe.* Simon and Schuster. 2008.

6　Albert Einstein. *Relativity: The Special and General Theory.* Penguin Classics. 2006.

7　George Gamow. *Gravity.* Dover. 2003.

8　James Gleick. *Genius: The Life and Science of Richard Feynman.* Vintage. 1993.

9　Richard Feynman. *QED: The Strange Theory of Light and Matter.* Princeton University Press. 2006.

10　Bertrand Russell. *History of Western Philosophy.* Routledge. 2004.

11　Simon Singh. *The Big Bang.* Harper Perennial. 2005.

12　Gerald Schroeder. *The Science of God: The Convergence of Scientific and Biblical Wisdom.* Broadway Books. 1998.

13　Homer (R. Fagles). *The Iliad.* Penguin Classics. 1998.

14　Richard Rhodes. *The Making of the Atomic Bomb.* Simon and Schuster. 1995.

15　Victor Hanson. *A War Like No Other: How the Athenians and Spartans Fought the Peloponnesian War.* Random House. 2006.

16　Thomas Cahill. *Sailing the Wine-Dark Sea: Why the Greeks Matter.* Anchor. 2004.

17　Michio Kaku. *Parallel Worlds: A Journey Through Creation, Higher Dimensions, and the Future of the Cosmos.* Anchor. 2006.

18　Gilbert Chesterton. *The Everlasting Man.* Wilder Publications. 2008.

19　Petr Beckmann. *A History of Pi.* St. Martin's Griffin. 1976.

20　Gary Taubes. *Good Calories, Bad Calories: Fats,*

Carbs, and the Controversial Science of Diet and Health. Anchor. 2008.

21 Victor Hanson. *Who Killed Homer? The Demise of Classical Education and the Recovery of Greek Wisdom.* Encounter Books. 2001.

22 Edwin Abbot. *Flatland: A Romance of Many Dimensions.* NuVision Publications. 2008.

23 Virgil (D. West). *The Aeneid.* Penguin Classics. 2003.

Index

For information on ordering additional copies of *The Relativity Diet: A Diet Theory of Everything*, please visit www.eventhorizonpublishing.com.